Praise for *Spastic Diplegia—Bilateral Cerebral Palsy*

"*After the success of the first edition of* Spastic Diplegia—Bilateral Cerebral Palsy, *it was time for Lily Collison and the team at Gillette to update their work. In this second edition, the text has been expanded with recent research summarized and referenced. The scope is comprehensive; the writing is clear. The journey the parents of a child with spastic diplegia embark on is frequently challenging and often frustrating due to the lack of a clear and authoritative 'user's guide.' Until the publication of this book, there was no single resource that parents could turn to for comprehensive and accurate information on a wide range of relevant topics. Here, every important aspect of spastic diplegia is addressed in a clear, conversational style that is faithful to the underlying research and science. I can think of no better guide for parents and families than this excellent text.*"

H. KERR GRAHAM, Professorial fellow, University of Melbourne; Honorary Consultant, The Royal Children's Hospital, Australia

"*The second edition of* Spastic Diplegia *is just as powerful if not more so than the first edition. I recommend this book to those with spastic diplegia and their families. It should also be required reading for anyone who is considering working in the CP field. This book will leave a lasting impact.*"

SAMANTHA MARIE LADEMANN, Student; Adult with spastic diplegia, US

"*Rarely does a book so comprehensively meet the needs of multiple stakeholders. The second edition of* Spastic Diplegia—Bilateral Cerebral Palsy *does just that. It is a reliable, rigorous, and incredibly readable summary of scientific and practical information about this condition. The generosity with which Lily and Tommy share their story, interwoven with facts about treatments, assessments, and aging, left me feeling reassured that great quality, usable information is available for people living with spastic diplegia. I highly recommend this book for both families and clinicians.*"

CATHY MORGAN, Principal Research Fellow and Program Lead Early Detection and Early Intervention, Cerebral Palsy Alliance Research Institute; Adjunct Associate Professor, Child and Adolescent Health, University of Sydney, Australia

"This book is an exceptional and comprehensive guide to understanding cerebral palsy in general and spastic diplegia in particular. It is a must-read for parents, caregivers, and family members of children and adults living with cerebral palsy. It covers a wide range of topics, including the causes, risk factors, diagnosis, classification, management, and treatment of the condition, in an informative and accessible manner. The inclusion of personal stories and tips from individuals and families living with spastic diplegia adds valuable insight into the lived experience of the condition. Overall, this book is an outstanding resource for families, medical professionals, and anyone seeking to gain a deeper understanding of spastic diplegia."

RACHEL THOMPSON, Co-Director, Southern Family Center for Cerebral Palsy, Rady Children's Hospital, San Diego; Associate Professor, Department of Orthopaedic Surgery, University of California, San Diego, US

"As a father to a teenager with cerebral palsy, as well as a scientist dedicated to understanding the unique health care needs facing individuals with cerebral palsy across the lifespan, I found this book to be an indispensable resource. There are very few options like this, which covers such a wide array of information that is relevant not only to spastic diplegia, but also to cerebral palsy as a general condition. I encourage any parent or caregiver of a child with cerebral palsy to consider this book as a guiding set of facts and recommendations pertaining to spastic diplegia and cerebral palsy in general."

MARK D. PETERSON, Professor, University of Michigan Medical School; Parent of a teenager with CP, US

"This book is an invaluable resource for families, empowering them with the knowledge and understanding they need to navigate a cerebral palsy diagnosis, the care, and the future. It also serves as an essential guide for health care professionals, providing comprehensive information crucial for delivering quality cerebral palsy care. As an orthopedic surgeon, I highly recommend it to both parents and medical practitioners. It should be considered mandatory reading for anyone dedicated to improving outcomes for individuals with cerebral palsy.

ENDA KELLY, Consultant Pediatric Orthopedic Surgeon, Children's Health Ireland

"Lily Collison and colleagues did an absolutely stunning job of writing this wonderful and thorough book that covers the many consequences of the complex disability of bilateral CP, and aging and living with it. The personal stories are moving and will be supportive for people with CP and their families; they also provide important insights to care providers. I hope this practical guide finds its way to parts of the world with less access to health care."

WILMA VAN DER SLOT, Rehabilitation physician and senior researcher, Rijndam Rehabilitation and Department of Rehabilitation Medicine, Erasmus MC, University Medical Center, Rotterdam, Netherlands

"*This is an indispensable guidebook for navigating spastic diplegia, as it is written for families with the condition. It imparts a deep understanding of the medical science and treatment pathways, supported by comprehensive evidence-based references and information resources. The author's generous sharing of her and her son's journey, and those of many others, provides valuable sign-posting, hope, and inspiration for the reader.*"

JEAN AND JOHN GLYNN, parents of a son with spastic diplegia, Ireland

"*This book is extremely well written. I have lived with spastic diplegia—bilateral cerebral palsy for almost 70 years, and yet I learned much from reading it. Each chapter focuses on a specific stage in the development of a person with spastic diplegic CP, from before birth to older adulthood. The author has done an excellent job of balancing the medical language and approach to addressing CP symptoms with the personal and family challenges associated with living with the condition. A particular strength of the book is the mother's ongoing narrative as her son, Tommy, progresses from his postnatal CP diagnosis through puberty, adolescence, and young adulthood, including the challenges faced at each stage and the medical procedures that were chosen to address these challenges. It definitely humanizes the clinical approach to CP interventions. This is a must-read for every member of the CP community, including individuals with CP and their family and caregivers, as well as professionals.*"

TED CONWAY, Research Professor, College of Engineering, Florida Atlantic University; Fellow, American Association for the Advancement of Science; Fellow, American Institute for Medical and Biological Engineering; Adult with spastic diplegia, US

"*This book is truly indispensable for a deeper understanding of the medical complexity and management of bilateral spastic diplegia from infancy to teen to adult, with both reliable medical information and valuable personal perspectives. With knowledge, we can comprehend, and that allows us to make the best informed decisions at a given point in time. As a parent, I have always wanted to know what the providers know about CP, but without medical training that is impossible. But armed with this clear and concise guide, my son and I can be an important part of the care conversation. It also honors the people with cerebral palsy and their caregivers by sharing their voices and wisdom. Brava to Lily Collison and the Gillette team for bringing this second edition to fruition!*"

LORI POLISKI, Parent of a young adult with spastic diplegia

"*This extremely useful resource for people with spastic diplegia and their families digests the current state-of-the-art care for children and adults in an organized and accessible format. The personal stories that accompany each section are poignant and informative. The book will be a great companion before and after medical visits as care decisions are being considered.*"

GAREY NORITZ, Director, Complex Health Care, Developmental and Behavioral Pediatrics, Nationwide Children's Hospital; Professor of Pediatrics, The Ohio State University; US

SPASTIC DIPLEGIA BILATERAL CEREBRAL PALSY

SPASTIC DIPLEGIA
Bilateral Cerebral Palsy

Second edition

Understanding and
managing the condition
across the lifespan:
A practical guide for families

Lily Collison, MA, MSc

Edited by
Jean Stout, PT, MS
Amy Schulz, PT, NCS
Candice Johnson, OTD, OTR/L
Tom F. Novacheck, MD
GILLETTE CHILDREN'S

Gillette Children's Healthcare Press
200 University Avenue East
St Paul, MN 55101
www.GilletteChildrensHealthcarePress.org
HealthcarePress@gillettechildrens.com

ISBN 978-1-952181-15-3 (paperback)
ISBN 978-1-952181-16-0 (e-book)
LIBRARY OF CONGRESS CONTROL NUMBER 2024941671

COPYEDITING BY Ruth Wilson
ORIGINAL ILLUSTRATIONS BY Olwyn Roche
COVER AND INTERIOR DESIGN BY Jazmin Welch
PROOFREADING BY Ruth Wilson
INDEX BY Audrey McClellan

Printed by Hobbs the Printers Ltd, Totton, Hampshire, UK

For information about distribution or special discounts for bulk purchases, please contact:
Mac Keith Press
2nd Floor, Rankin Building
139-143 Bermondsey Street
London, SE1 3UW
www.mackeith.co.uk
admin@mackeith.co.uk

To individuals and families whose lives are affected by these conditions, to professionals who serve our community, and to all clinicians and researchers who push the knowledge base forward, we hope the books in this Healthcare Series serve you very well.

Gillette Children's acknowledges a grant from the Cerebral Palsy Foundation for the writing of this book.

All proceeds from the books in this series at Gillette Children's go to research.

Contents

APPENDICES (ONLINE)

Author and Editors

Lily Collison, MA, MSc, Program Director, Gillette Children's Healthcare Press

Jean Stout, PT, MS, PhDc, Research Physical Therapist, James R. Gage Center for Gait and Motion Analysis, Gillette Children's

Amy Schulz, PT, NCS, Physical Therapist and Clinical Educator, Gillette Children's

Candice Johnson, OTD, OTR/L, Rehabilitation Therapies Administrative Supervisor–CORE (Clinical Outcomes, Research, and Education), Gillette Children's and Gillette Phalen Clinic

Tom F. Novacheck, MD, Medical Director of Integrated Care Services, Gillette Children's; Professor of Orthopedics, University of Minnesota; and Past President, American Academy for Cerebral Palsy and Developmental Medicine

Series Foreword

You hold in your hands one book in the Gillette Children's Healthcare Series. This series was inspired by multiple factors.

It started with Lily Collison writing the first book in the series, *Spastic Diplegia–Bilateral Cerebral Palsy*. Lily has a background in medical science and is the parent of a now adult son who has spastic diplegia. Lily was convincing at the time about the value of such a book, and with the publication of that book in 2020, Gillette Children's became one of the first children's hospitals in the world to set up its own publishing arm—Gillette Children's Healthcare Press. *Spastic Diplegia–Bilateral Cerebral Palsy* received very positive reviews from both families and professionals and achieved strong sales. Unsolicited requests came in from diverse organizations across the globe for translation rights, and feedback from families told us there was a demand for books relevant to other conditions.

We listened.

We were convinced of the value of expanding from one book into a series to reflect Gillette Children's strong commitment to worldwide education. In 2021, Lily joined the press as Program Director, and very quickly, Gillette Children's formed teams to write the Healthcare Series. The series includes, in order of publication:

- *Craniosynostosis*
- *Idiopathic Scoliosis*
- *Spastic Hemiplegia—Unilateral Cerebral Palsy*
- *Spastic Quadriplegia—Bilateral Cerebral Palsy*
- *Spastic Diplegia—Bilateral Cerebral Palsy, second edition*
- *Epilepsy*
- *Spina Bifida*
- *Osteogenesis Imperfecta*
- *Scoliosis—Congenital, Neuromuscular, Syndromic, and Other Causes*

The books address each condition detailing both the medical and human story.

Mac Keith Press, long-time publisher of books on disability and the journal *Developmental Medicine and Child Neurology,* is co-publishing this series with Gillette Children's Healthcare Press.

Families and professionals working well together is key to best management of any condition. The parent is the expert of their child while the professional is the expert of the condition. These books underscore the importance of that family and professional partnership. For each title in the series, medical professionals at Gillette Children's have led the writing, and families contributed the lived experience.

These books have been written in the United States with an international lens and citing international research. However, there isn't always strong evidence to create consensus in medicine, so others may take a different view.

We hope you find the book you hold in your hands to be of great value. We collectively strive to optimize outcomes for children, adolescents, and adults living with these childhood-acquired and largely lifelong conditions.

Dr. Tom F. Novacheck

Series Introduction

The Healthcare Series seeks to optimize outcomes for those who live with childhood-acquired physical and/or neurological conditions. The conditions addressed in this series of books are complex and often have many associated challenges. Although the books focus on the biomedical aspects of each condition, we endeavor to address each condition as holistically as possible. Since the majority of people with these conditions have them for life, the life course is addressed including transition and aging issues.

Who are these books for?

These books are written for an international audience. They are primarily written for parents of young children, but also for adolescents and adults who have the condition. They are written for members of multidisciplinary teams and researchers. Finally, they are written for others, including extended family members, teachers, and students taking courses in the fields of medicine, allied health care, and education.

A worldview

The books in the series focus on evidence-based best practice, which we acknowledge is not available everywhere. It is mostly available in high-income countries (at least in urban areas, though even there, not always), but many families live away from centers of good care.

We also acknowledge that the majority of people with disabilities live in low- and middle-income countries. Improving the lives of all those with disabilities across the globe is an important goal. Developing scalable, affordable interventions is a crucial step toward achieving this. Nonetheless, the best interventions will fail if we do not first address the social determinants of health—the economic, social, and environmental conditions in which people live that shape their overall health and well-being.

No family reading these books should ever feel they have failed their child. We all struggle to do our best for our children within the limitations of our various resources and situations. Indeed, the advocacy role these books may play may help families and professionals lobby in unison for best care.

International Classification of Functioning, Disability and Health

The writing of the series of books has been informed by the International Classification of Functioning, Disability and Health (ICF).[1] The framework explains the impact of a health condition at different levels and how those levels are interconnected. It tells us to look at the full picture—to look at the person with a disability in their life situation.

The framework shows that every human being can experience a decrease in health and thereby experience some disability. It is not something that happens only to a minority of people. The ICF thus "mainstreams" disability and recognizes it as a widespread human experience.

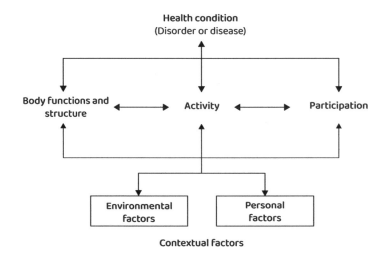

International Classification of Functioning, Disability and Health (ICF). Reproduced with kind permission from WHO.

In health care, there has been a shift away from focusing almost exclusively on correcting issues that cause the individual's functional problems to focusing also on the individual's activity and participation. These books embrace maximizing participation for all people living with disability.

The Family

For simplicity, throughout the series we refer to "parents" and "children"; we acknowledge, however, that family structures vary. "Parent" is used as a generic term that includes grandparents, relatives, and carers (caregivers) who are raising a child. Throughout the series, we refer to male and female as the biologic sex assigned at birth. We acknowledge that this does not equate to gender identity or sexual orientation, and we respect the individuality of each person. Throughout the series we have included both "person with disability" and "disabled person," recognizing that both terms are used.

Caring for a child with a disability can be challenging and overwhelming. Having a strong social support system in place can make a difference. For the parent, balancing the needs of the child with a disability with the needs of siblings—while also meeting employment demands, nurturing a relationship with a significant other, and caring for aging parents—can sometimes feel like an enormous juggling act. Siblings may feel neglected or overlooked because of the increased attention given to the disabled child. It is crucial for parents to allocate time and resources to ensure that siblings feel valued and included in the family dynamics. Engaging siblings in the care and support of the disabled child can help foster a sense of unity and empathy within the family.

A particular challenge for a child and adolescent who has a disability, and their parent, is balancing school attendance (for both academic and social purposes) with clinical appointments and surgery. Appointments outside of school hours are encouraged. School is important because the cognitive and social abilities developed there help maximize employment opportunities when employment is a realistic goal. Indeed, technology has eliminated barriers and created opportunities that did not exist even 10 years ago.

Parents also need to find a way to prioritize self-care. Neglecting their own well-being can have detrimental effects on their mental and physical health. Think of the safety advice on an airplane: you are told that you must put on your own oxygen mask before putting on your child's. It's the same when caring for a child with a disability; parents need to take care of themselves in order to effectively care for their child *and* family. Friends, support groups, or mental health professionals can provide an outlet for parents to express their emotions, gain valuable insights, and find solace in knowing that they are not alone in their journey.

For those of you reading this book who have the condition, we hope this book gives you insights into its many nuances and complexities, acknowledges you as an expert in your own care, and provides a road map and framework for you to advocate for your needs.

Last words

This series of books seeks to be an invaluable educational resource. All proceeds from the series at Gillette Children's go to research.

Chapter 1

Cerebral palsy

Introduction

So be sure when you step.
Step with care and great tact
and remember that Life's
a Great Balancing Act …
And will you succeed?
Yes! You will, indeed!
(98 and ¾ percent guaranteed.)
Kid, you'll move mountains!

Dr. Seuss

To fully understand spastic diplegia, it is worth first having an understanding of the umbrella term "cerebral palsy" (CP). "Cerebral" refers to a specific part of the brain (the cerebrum) and "palsy" literally means paralysis (cerebrum paralysis). Although paralysis describes something different from the typical features of CP, it is the origin of the term "palsy."

CP was first described in 1861 by an English doctor, William Little, and for many years it was known as "Little's disease." Over the years there has been much discussion of the definition of CP, and different definitions have been adopted and later discarded. Following is the most recently adopted definition, published in 2007:

> Cerebral palsy describes a group of permanent disorders of the development of movement and posture, causing activity limitation, that are attributed to non-progressive disturbances that occurred in the developing fetal or infant brain. The motor disorders of cerebral palsy are often accompanied by disturbances of sensation, perception, cognition, communication, behaviour, by epilepsy and by secondary musculoskeletal problems.[2]

In other words, CP is a *group* of conditions caused by an injury to the developing brain, which can result in a variety of motor and other problems that affect how the child functions. Because the injury occurs in a *developing brain and growing child*, problems often change over time, even though the brain injury itself is unchanging. Table 1.1.1 explains the terms used in the definition of CP above, in order.

Table 1.1.1 Explanation of terms in definition of CP

TERMS	EXPLANATION
Cerebral	"Cerebral" refers to the cerebrum, one of the major areas of the brain responsible for the control of movement.
Palsy	"Palsy" means paralysis, that is, an inability to activate muscles by the nervous system, though paralysis by pure definition is not a feature of CP.
Group	CP is not a single condition, unlike conditions such as type 1 diabetes. Rather, CP is a group of conditions. The location, timing, and type of brain injury vary, as do the resulting effects.
Permanent	The brain injury remains for life; CP is a permanent, lifelong condition.
Disorders	A disorder is a disruption in the usual orderly process. To meet the definition of CP, the disorder must cause activity limitation.
Posture	Posture is the way a person holds their body when, for example, standing, sitting, or moving.

Cont'd.

TERMS	EXPLANATION
Activity limitation	An activity is the execution of a task or action by an individual. Activity limitations are difficulties an individual may have in doing activities. Walking with difficulty is an example.
Nonprogressive	The brain injury does not worsen, but its effects can develop or evolve over time.
Developing fetal or infant brain	The brain of a fetus or infant has not finished developing all its neural connections and is therefore immature. An injury to an immature brain is different from an injury to a mature brain.
Motor disorders	Motor disorders are conditions affecting the ability to move and the quality of those movements.
Sensation	"Sensation" can be defined as a physical feeling or perception arising from something that happens to or that comes in contact with the body.
Perception	Perception is the ability to incorporate and interpret sensory and/or cognitive information.
Cognition	"Cognition" means the mental action or process of acquiring knowledge and understanding through thought, experience, and the senses.
Communication	Communication is the imparting or exchanging of information.
Behavior	"Behavior" refers to the way a person acts or conducts themselves.
Epilepsy	Epilepsy is a neurological disorder in which brain electrical activity becomes abnormal, causing seizures or periods of unusual behavior, sensations, and sometimes loss of awareness.
Secondary musculoskeletal problems	"Musculoskeletal" refers to both the muscles and the skeleton (i.e., the muscles, bones, joints, and their related structures). Musculoskeletal problems appear with time and growth and are therefore termed "secondary problems." They develop as a consequence of the brain injury. People with CP may develop a variety of musculoskeletal problems, such as bone torsion (twist), or muscle contracture (a limitation of range of motion of a joint).

Adapted from Rosenbaum and colleagues.[2]

CP is the most common cause of physical disability in children.[3] It is acquired during pregnancy, birth, or in early childhood, and it is a lifelong condition. There is currently no cure, nor is one imminent, but good management and treatment (addressed in Chapter 3) can help alleviate some or many of the effects of the brain injury.

When the brain injury occurs is important. The consequences of a brain injury to a fetus developing in the uterus are generally different from those of a brain injury sustained at birth, which in turn are different from those of a brain injury acquired during infancy. The European and Australian Cerebral Palsy Registers use two years of age as the cutoff for applying the diagnosis of CP.[4,5] A brain injury occurring after two years of age is called an "acquired brain injury." This two-year cutoff is applied because of the differences in brain maturity relative to when the brain injury occurs.

Although the development of movement and posture is affected in individuals with CP, as seen above, other body systems can also be affected.

How to read this book

To help you navigate the information in this book, it has been organized so that you can read it from beginning to end or, alternatively, dip into different sections and chapters independently. Because much of the information builds on previous sections and chapters, it is best to first read the book in its entirety to get an overall sense of the condition. After that, you can return to the parts that are relevant to you, knowing that you can ignore other sections or revisit them if and when they do become relevant.

This chapter addresses the overall condition of CP. Chapter 2 addresses spastic diplegia, and Chapter 3 covers the management of treatment of spastic diplegia to age 20. Chapter 4 looks at spastic diplegia in adulthood.

Throughout Chapters 1 to 4, medical information is interspersed with personal lived experience. Orange boxes are used to highlight the personal story. Chapter 5 is devoted to vignettes from individuals and families around the globe. Chapter 6 provides further reading and research.

At the back of the book, you'll find a glossary of key terms.

A companion website for this book is available at www.GilletteChildrens HealthcarePress.org. This website contains some useful web resources and appendices. A QR code to access **Useful web resources** is included below.

It may be helpful to discuss any questions you may have from reading this book with your medical professional.

My third son, Tommy, was born at term in Ireland in 1994. His older brothers, then aged four and six, had been easy babies, so by then my husband and I felt quite relaxed as parents. Tommy was born after an uneventful pregnancy and delivery, but from birth he cried incessantly. At three weeks, our family physician insisted that I give up breastfeeding. She could see how frazzled I had become due to Tommy's constant crying, his difficulty with feeding (many feeds were being returned), and the fact that neither he nor I was getting much sleep.

At three months the incessant crying suddenly stopped; Tommy became a serene, happy, and placid child, and we all relaxed again. However, a few months later, at a routine developmental check, he was deemed "developmentally delayed." That started a long journey, beginning with the diagnosis of spastic diplegia when he was a year old and continuing with the management and treatment of his condition in our community as well as at the Central Remedial Clinic* in Dublin. In the early years he also received conductive education,† and in adolescence he had a number of surgeries at Gillette Children's in Minnesota.

At the time of writing, Tommy, now 30 years old, is a college graduate, working full time, married, and living an independent life in the US.

---

* Then, a national treatment center for people with physical disabilities.

† Conductive education is based on an educational rather than a medical model for treatment of children with CP. It combines educational and rehabilitation goals into a single program.

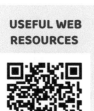

USEFUL WEB RESOURCES

The nervous system

The Brain—is wider than the Sky
Emily Dickinson

CP results from an injury to the developing fetal or young child's brain, or a difference in how the fetal brain forms. A basic understanding of the nervous system is useful to help understand the effects of the brain injury. This section briefly explains the main components of the nervous system.

The nervous system is composed of the:

- Central nervous system (CNS)—the brain and spinal cord.
- Peripheral nervous system (PNS)—a large network of nerves that carry messages between the CNS and the rest of the body. The autonomic nervous system is part of the PNS; it controls involuntary functions of the brain and body, such as breathing, heart rate, and digestion.

See Figure 1.2.1.

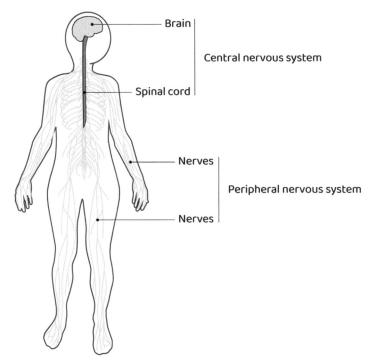

Figure 1.2.1 The nervous system.

Nerve cells

The nerve cell (also known as "neuron" or "neurone") is the basic unit of the nervous system. Nerve cells carry information between the CNS and the rest of the body as electrical impulses. There are three types of nerve cells:

- Motor nerve cells, which take information from the CNS to a muscle or gland
- Sensory nerve cells, which do the opposite, taking messages from the rest of the body to the CNS
- Interneurons (also known as "relay neurons"), which carry information between nerve cells

Figure 1.2.2 shows a typical nerve cell. Note the cell body and axon. Information enters the nerve cell through the dendrites and cell body, and exits via the axonal endings. The cell bodies form the gray matter of the brain, and the axons form the white matter, or the communication tracts.

The whitish color of the white matter is due to the fatty substance, called "myelin," that covers the axons; this insulates and speeds up the transmission of electrical impulses. Nerve cells receive, interpret, and transfer messages as electrical impulses. These electrical impulses form the brain's electrical activity, which can be measured and recorded on an electroencephalogram (EEG).

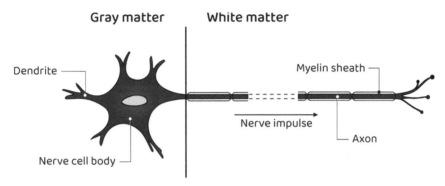

Figure 1.2.2 Nerve cell. Adapted with kind permission from *The Identification and Treatment of Gait Problems in Cerebral Palsy*, 2nd edition, edited by James Gage et al. (2009). Mac Keith Press.

Brain structure and functions

The brain is housed inside the cranium, a bony covering that protects the brain from external injury. Together, the cranium and the bones that protect the face make up the skull.

The brain is divided into several distinct parts that serve important functions. See Figure 1.2.3.

The *cerebrum* is the front and upper part of the brain. The cerebral cortex (the outer layer, the surface of the brain) is the gray matter where the cell bodies of the nerve cells are found. The cerebral cortex has a large surface area and, due to its folds, it appears wrinkled. Different regions of the cerebral cortex have different functions.

The *cerebellum* is located at the back of the brain, under the cerebrum, and helps with maintaining balance and posture, coordination, and fine motor movements.

The *brain stem* is the bottom part of the brain that connects the cerebrum to the *spinal cord*. It also serves as a relay station for messages between different parts of the body and the cerebral cortex. Many functions responsible for survival are located here (e.g., breathing and heart rate).

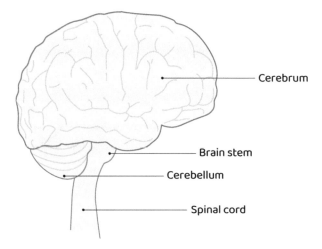

Figure 1.2.3 Parts of the brain.

The cerebrum is divided in two halves, referred to as hemispheres (see Figure 1.2.4). In general, the right half controls the left side of the body, and the left half controls the right side of the body. Therefore, damage on the right side of the cerebrum will impact the left side of the body and vice versa. Communication between the two halves occurs in the corpus callosum, located in the center of the cerebrum.

The *basal ganglia* and *thalamus* are located in the middle of the cerebrum, deep beneath the cerebral cortex. The basal ganglia are important in the control of movement, including motor learning and planning. The thalamus is sometimes referred to as a relay station—it relays various sensory information (e.g., sight, sound, touch) to the cerebral cortex from the rest of the body.

Cerebrospinal fluid is found within the brain and around the spinal cord. It is produced within channels in the brain, called ventricles. Cerebrospinal fluid helps protect the brain and spinal cord from injury.

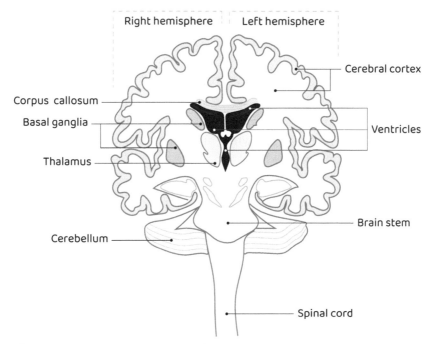

Right hemisphere | Left hemisphere

Corpus callosum

Basal ganglia

Thalamus

Cerebellum

Cerebral cortex

Ventricles

Brain stem

Spinal cord

Figure 1.2.4 Vertical cross-section of the brain.

The term "cerebral palsy" first came into our lives when Tommy was about one year old. Until then, it was a term I was vaguely familiar with but could not have explained.

Tommy missed developmental milestones and was initially described as "developmentally delayed." Months passed, but no diagnosis was forthcoming. By his first birthday, he was unable to sit without support or even hold a bottle. I decided to seek a second opinion from a pediatrician known to be a straight talker. On the day of the appointment, I collected our two older children from school. They remained in the waiting room, happy with the promise of a visit to the McDonald's next door after the appointment.

After the usual brief introductory pleasantries, the pediatrician examined Tommy. The conversation that followed went something like this:

Pediatrician: Do you not know what's wrong with this child?

Me: (*Politely*) No. (*Thinking*: If I did, I wouldn't be here.)

Pediatrician: (*Matter-of-fact*) He has cerebral palsy. And what's more, if I want to know how this child will turn out, I don't look at the child, I look at the mother.

Though this was certainly not what I had expected, nor what I wanted to hear, I felt a strange sense of relief after the months of uncertainty and worry. I appreciated knowing and I appreciated the doctor's straight-talking manner.

That day, three lively children and one dazed mother visited McDonald's. That day, I had no opinion on the matter, but now, almost 30 years later, I definitely agree with the pediatrician: we parents are key influencers of outcome. That day, having received Tommy's diagnosis, I wish I could have been given this book.

Causes, risk factors, and prevalence

The little reed, bending to the force of the wind, soon
stood upright again when the storm had passed over.

Aesop

The US Centers for Disease Control and Prevention (CDC) defines
"cause" as:

> *A factor (characteristic, behavior, event, etc.) that directly influences the occurrence of disease. A reduction of the factor in the population should lead to a reduction in the occurrence of disease.*

It defines "risk factor" as:

> *An aspect of personal behavior or lifestyle, an environmental exposure, or an inborn or inherited characteristic that is associated with an increased occurrence of disease or other health-related event or condition.*[6]

Causes thus have a stronger relationship with CP than do risk factors.
A significant stroke in the infant's brain, for example, is a cause of CP.

Preterm birth (i.e., less than 37 weeks gestation) is a risk factor but not a cause of CP—in other words, not every preterm infant is found to have CP. There are many possible causes of brain injury, including events during fetal development, pregnancy, birth, or early infant life. Much is known about the causes and risk factors for CP, but more remains unknown.

Causes

Data from Australia shows that 94 percent of children with CP had a brain injury in the prenatal or perinatal periods (i.e., during pregnancy and up to the first 28 days after birth), while only 6 percent had a recognized postnatal brain injury (acquired more than 28 days after birth and before two years of age).[4] Seventy to 80 percent of CP cases are associated with prenatal factors, and birth asphyxia (lack of oxygen during birth) plays a relatively minor role.[7]

There are many causes of brain injury, including:

- **Hypoxia-ischemia:** from hypoxia, which is a deficiency of oxygen, and ischemia, which is reduced blood flow to the brain. Hypoxia-ischemia is a combination of both terms
- **Hemorrhage:** bleeding in the brain, also termed a "cerebral vascular accident" (CVA) or a stroke
- **Infection**
- **Abnormalities in brain development**[7]

A decrease in oxygen and insufficient blood supply to the brain have different effects in preterm infants compared with term infants due to the different stages of their brain development. As noted in section 1.2, the nerve cell bodies form the gray matter while axons form the white matter or the communication tracts. It has been found that white matter injuries predominate in infants born preterm, whereas gray matter injuries are more common in infants born at term.[7]

Approximately 90 percent of cases of CP result from healthy brain tissue becoming damaged rather than from abnormalities in brain development.[3] The cause of CP in an individual child is very often unknown.[8,9]

Risk Factors

Infants who are born preterm (earlier than 37 weeks) or who have low birth weight have a higher risk of CP.[10] Twins and other multiple-birth siblings are at particular risk because they tend to be born early and at lower birth weights. Australian data shows that:[4]

- Forty-three percent of births of children with CP were preterm compared to 9 percent in the typical population.
- Forty-three percent of children with CP were born with low birth weight (under 2,500 grams, or 5.5 lb) compared to 7 percent in the typical population.
- The prevalence of children with CP was higher for twin than singleton births. This is why single embryo transfer in assisted reproductive technology (ART)* is strongly encouraged.[11,12]

In addition to the above, other risk factors for CP include the following (not an exhaustive list):[7]

- Prior to conception:
  - Young or advanced maternal age
  - A history of stillbirth or multiple miscarriages
  - Low socioeconomic status
  - Genetic factors
- During pregnancy:
  - Male sex: Males account for a greater proportion of individuals with CP than females. Australia data shows that 58 percent of those with CP were male.[4]
  - TORCH complex: TORCH is an acronym used to refer to a group of infections that can affect a developing fetus or a newborn: **T**oxoplasmosis (caused by a parasite), **O**ther infections, **R**ubella (also known as German measles), **C**ytomegalovirus, and **H**erpes simplex virus.
  - Maternal thyroid disorder.
  - Pre-eclampsia (high blood pressure that can pose serious risks to both mother and fetus if left untreated).

---

* A broad term encompassing various fertility treatments, including in vitro fertilization, intrauterine insemination, and egg freezing.

- ○   Placenta problems (e.g., placenta previa, placenta abruption).[*]
- Around the time of birth and during the neonatal (newborn) period:
  - ○   An acute hypoxic event (lack of oxygen) during birth
  - ○   Meconium aspiration[†]
  - ○   Seizures
  - ○   Low blood sugar

Some risk factors are declining, but others are increasing. Although any one risk factor may cause CP, if that factor is severe enough, it is more often caused by the combination of multiple risk factors.[13] Although preterm birth is a large risk factor for CP, it's the causal pathways that have led to it, or the consequences of it, that may cause the CP, rather than the preterm birth itself.

Mutations or changes in the genes involved in brain development or function (either inherited or *de novo,* which is a change in a gene that appears for the first time in a child but is not present in either parent) can increase susceptibility to CP. These genetic risk factors may affect the severity of symptoms, the specific type of CP, or the likelihood of associated conditions. Genetic risk factors may interact with other risk factors, highlighting the complex interplay between multiple risk factors in determining the development of the condition.

In low- and middle-income countries, causes and risk factors differ. In these countries, few preterm infants survive. Birth asphyxia is more common due to complications during labor or delivery. Also more common is Rhesus incompatibility (a mismatch in the Rhesus blood group system between the mother and the fetus). As well, a higher proportion of postnatally acquired CP is associated with infections such as meningitis, septicemia, and malaria.[7]

---

[*] "Placenta previa" means the placenta partially or fully covers the cervix. It can lead to bleeding and complications during birth. "Placenta abruption" means the placenta detaches from the uterus before the infant is born, with potentially life-threatening risks for both the mother and infant. It requires immediate medical attention.

[†] When a newborn breathes in a mixture of amniotic fluid (fluid that was surrounding the fetus in the uterus) and stool during or shortly after birth, potentially causing respiratory issues.

> We don't know what caused Tommy's CP, but that is not unusual. Like many other parents, I would like to have known.

Prevalence

The prevalence of a condition is how many people in a defined population have the condition at a specific point in time. Prevalence can vary geographically and change over time because of medical advances and social and economic development.

Having an understanding of prevalence, along with causes and risk factors, can help with prevention of CP. A systematic review* of interventions for prevention and treatment of CP reported that effective prenatal interventions include corticosteroids and magnesium sulfate; effective neonatal (newborn) interventions include caffeine (methylxanthine) and hypothermia.†[14]

CP registers‡ are essential for tracking and analyzing the prevalence and trends of CP in populations. They provide researchers and health care providers with critical data on the incidence, types, severity, and outcomes of CP, which can lead to improved health care policies and practices. It would be very helpful if, once a child is diagnosed with CP, parents would give consent to have their child added to a CP register.

Many countries maintain CP registers. There are two major networks of registers: the Surveillance of Cerebral Palsy in Europe (SCPE, established in 1998) and the Australian Cerebral Palsy Register (ACPR, established in 2007). A newer network of registers was established in 2018: the Global Low- and Middle-Income Countries CP Register (GLM CPR). There is no single national CP register in the US. There, instead, CP data is often collected and maintained by various state or regional programs, research facilities, or health care centers.

---

* A systematic review summarizes the results of a number of scientific studies.

† The controlled cooling of a newborn's body temperature.[20]

‡ Confidential databases that store important data about individuals with CP.

The current CP birth prevalence in high-income countries is declining and is now 1.6 per 1,000 live births (data 1995 to 2014).[5] However, in the US, prevalence was found to be higher at 2.9 per 1,000 eight-year-olds (2010 data)[15] and 3.2 per 1,000 3- to 17-year-olds (2009–2016 data).[16]

Current CP birth prevalence is also higher in low- and middle-income countries.[5] The prevalence in rural Bangladesh was reported as 3.4 per 1,000 children, and the majority had potentially preventable risk factors.[17] For example, only 30 percent of mothers received regular prenatal care.[17]

The most recent report from the Australian Cerebral Palsy Register shows a decrease in both prevalence and severity of CP between 1997 and 2016.[4] The decrease in prevalence was from 2.4 to 1.5 per 1,000 live births, a decrease of almost 40 percent. The decrease in severity was evidenced by a decrease in the proportion of children with greater functional mobility challenges, and in the proportion of children with epilepsy or intellectual impairment. This is encouraging because it suggests that with the application of resources, prevalence and severity may be able to be reduced in other countries.

Unfortunately, funding for CP research is very low. Although the reported prevalence of CP is double that of Down syndrome,[18] funding awarded for CP research in 2023 ($30 million) was significantly lower than for Down syndrome research ($133 million).[19]

Though I did not know what caused Tommy's CP, in the early days I wasted a lot of time feeling guilty. I had worked very hard and was stressed during his pregnancy, and I felt responsible. Today, I no longer feel that sense of guilt. I didn't knowingly do anything wrong: my life circumstances were such that I was very busy, and besides, there are multiple possible causes of brain injury. I encourage parents to waste no time on guilt—we are where we are and we move forward.

Diagnosis

Acceptance is knowing that grief is a raging river. And you have to get into it. Because when you do, it carries you to the next place. It eventually takes you to open land, somewhere where it will turn out OK in the end.

Simone George

There is no single test to confirm CP, unlike other conditions such as type 1 diabetes, which is confirmed through a simple blood test for glucose, or Down syndrome, which is confirmed through a genetic test. Recall that CP is not a single condition; rather, it is a group of conditions. The location, timing, and type of brain injury vary, and the resulting effects of the brain injury are also varied.

Until recently, a diagnosis of CP was generally made between 12 and 24 months based on a combination of clinical signs (e.g., lack of use of a limb), neurological symptoms (e.g., presence of spasticity*), and physical limitations (e.g., delayed independent sitting or walking). However,

---

* A condition in which there is an abnormal increase in muscle tone or stiffness of muscle that can interfere with movement and speech, and be associated with discomfort or pain.[22]

using certain standardized tests in combination with clinical examination and medical history, Novak and colleagues found that a diagnosis of CP can often accurately be made before six months corrected age.[*][21] They identified two distinct pathways in their International Clinical Practice Guideline for early diagnosis of CP:

- Before five months corrected age, for infants with newborn detectable risk factors (e.g., preterm):
  - MRI (magnetic resonance imaging)
  - GMs (Prechtl Qualitative Assessment of General Movements)[†]
  - HINE (Hammersmith Infant Neurological Examination)[‡]
- After five months corrected age for infants with infant detectable risk factors (e.g., delayed motor milestones)
  - MRI
  - HINE
  - DAYC (Developmental Assessment of Young Children)[§]

The presence of a brain injury is confirmed by MRI in many but not all children with CP. Imaging may also help determine when the brain injury occurred.[3] However, up to 17 percent of children diagnosed with CP have normal MRI brain scans.[3] For these children, best practice is to investigate further to rule out genetic and metabolic conditions.[3]

Successful implementation of early diagnosis programs has been demonstrated in different countries.[23-28] Early diagnosis is very important because it allows for early intervention, which helps to achieve better functional outcomes for the child.

---

* The term "corrected age" refers to how old an infant would be if they had been born on their due date rather than preterm. "Chronological age" refers to how old an infant is from their date of birth. Corrected age is often used when assessing growth and developmental skills usually up to a chronological age of two years. With preterm infants, it takes time to determine whether the delays are related to being preterm or are true delays.

† A standardized assessment of movement for infants, from birth to five months corrected age. It involves a video of an infant lying on their back while they are awake, calm, and alert. The recorded movements are then scored by a certified medical professional.

‡ A standardized neurological examination for infants age 2 to 24 months performed by a medical professional. There are three parts to the exam: carrying out a neurological examination (which is scored), noting developmental milestones, and observing behavior (both not scored).

§ A standardized assessment for infants and children from birth to five years, in which a medical professional scores a child's skills during observation of play or daily activity, asking a child to perform a skill, or by interviewing parents to measure ability in five domains: cognition, communication, social-emotional development, physical development, and adaptive behavior.

Where a CP diagnosis is suspected but cannot be made with certainty, using the interim diagnosis of "high risk for CP" is recommended until a diagnosis is confirmed.[29] This allows the child to receive the benefits of CP-specific early intervention.[30]

These early interventions are designed to:[21]

- Optimize motor, cognition, and communication skills using interventions that promote learning and neuroplasticity
- Prevent secondary impairments and minimize complications that worsen function or interfere with learning (e.g., monitor hips, control epilepsy, take care of sleeping, feeding)
- Promote parent or caregiver coping and mental health

Neuroplasticity (also known as brain plasticity, neural plasticity, and neuronal plasticity) refers to the brain's ability to change. After a brain injury occurs, the brain will try to recover somewhat by creating new pathways around the injury, moving functions to a healthy area of the brain, or strengthening existing healthy connections. This potential for change and growth through practice and repetition allows the brain to develop new skills.[31,32]

Neuroplasticity is at its optimum during early brain development. The first thousand days are a critical time for brain development; this is a time when interventions are particularly effective.[33] This is also a time of extreme vulnerability: the same neuroplasticity that gives a child the potential to recover function also makes them very sensitive to any intervention, which can result in unwanted consequences unless the intervention has been proven safe.

Morgan and colleagues published an International Clinical Practice Guideline for early intervention for children from birth to two years of age with or at high risk of CP.[30] They followed this with another guideline in 2023 for children in the first year of life, which helps determine the most appropriate motor intervention to implement.[34]

These clinical practice guidelines for early diagnosis and early intervention should become standard of care[21,30,34] and be continually updated. The advancements in early diagnosis have resulted in multiple clinical trials in early interventions around the world, which will add to the research base in the coming years. (Further information on clinical trials is included in Chapter 6.)

Graham and colleagues noted that mothers of children with CP who have previously had a typically developing child often sense that something is wrong at a very early stage; they advised professionals to take the concerns of an experienced parent seriously.[3] Indeed, "parent-identified concern" is included in the International Clinical Practice Guideline for early diagnosis as a "valid reason to trigger formal diagnostic investigations and referral to early intervention."[21] Parent focus groups have also found that receiving early diagnosis or high risk for CP classification is a parent priority.[35]

Emily Perl Kingsley, who was a writer on the TV show *Sesame Street*, wrote a short essay titled "Welcome to Holland" in 1987 about parenting her son, born with Down syndrome. She described it as going on vacation and arriving at a different destination than what was expected. The essay resonates with many families on receiving a diagnosis of CP and is included in **Useful web resources**.

Receiving the news that your beautiful child has CP is very tough for parents, who may then go through a grieving process. Looking back, I found that the diagnosis was almost a help after all the months of uncertainty. It galvanized me into immediate action to find out how I could best help my child. This was probably my way of coping with the news. Every parent will deal with the diagnosis in their own way, but I would encourage all parents to try to get as good an understanding of the condition as they can, as soon as they can. To that end, this book may be helpful.

Looking back at photographs from Tommy's first year, I can now see that the signs of his CP were obvious from very early on. In retrospect, I feel his diagnosis could have been made much earlier. Because he wasn't diagnosed until he was a year old, intervention only started in earnest then. If a clinician suspects a child of having CP, I believe they should communicate this to the parents immediately. The possible harm done by delaying diagnosis, and therefore intervention, is to my mind greater than the possible harm done by raising a suspicion that later proves unwarranted. The only intervention the child is likely to receive during that period is therapies, which won't do them any harm.

What should a medical professional (e.g., a therapist) who is not responsible for diagnosis do if they strongly suspect a child in their care has CP? In my view, such a professional has a responsibility to communicate, without delay, with the person responsible for diagnosis. Likewise, if parents have any suspicion that their child may have a problem, they should communicate it to their physician as soon as possible.

I sensed that something was wrong when Tommy was just a day old. He cried so incessantly that by evening I asked if he could be checked by a pediatrician. I did not feel all was fine; his prolonged crying had an unusual pitch. The on-duty pediatrician came to see him and reassured me that all was well, and I accepted her reassurance. Years later, I remember gently suggesting to a close friend that she have her baby assessed because I felt he had a very unusual cry. My friend's baby turned out to have a significant intellectual disability.

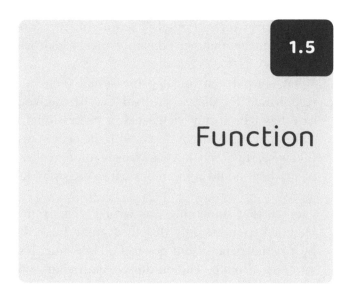

1.5

Function

That's one small step for man, one giant leap for mankind.
Neil Armstrong

"Function" means ability or capacity. "Motor function" refers to our ability to move, and "communication function" refers to our ability to transmit and receive information by whatever means. CP affects the development of movement, but it can also affect other areas, such as cognition. This section introduces the broad area of function and, again, lays groundwork for later sections.

Developmental milestones

The CDC published a series of developmental milestones that address typical development of the child from the age of two months to five years, in the following areas:[36]

- Social/emotional
- Language/communication

- Cognitive
- Movement/physical development

These milestones are an important reference when a child appears to be late in development compared with typically developing children. The CDC developmental milestones are included in **Useful web resources**.

Movement and physical development depend on the development and maturation of gross and fine motor function.

- **Gross motor function** (or gross motor skills): the movement of the arms, legs, and other large body parts. It involves the use of large muscles. Examples include sitting, crawling, standing, running, jumping, swimming, throwing, catching, and kicking. These movements involve maintaining balance and changing position.
- **Fine motor function** (or fine motor skills, hand skills, fine motor coordination, or dexterity): the smaller movements that occur in the wrists, hands, fingers, feet, and toes. It involves the control of small muscles. Examples include picking up objects between the thumb and forefinger, and writing. These movements typically involve hand-eye coordination and require a high degree of precision of hand and finger movement.

There is a usual sequence and timing to the achievement of gross motor developmental milestones in the typically developing child. A large study conducted by the World Health Organization (WHO) found that, with some variation, almost all typically developing children have achieved independent sitting by 9 months and independent walking by 18 months.[37] The average age and age range for achieving each of six gross motor developmental milestones are shown in Figure 1.5.1.

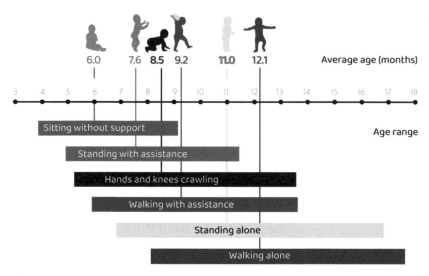

Figure 1.5.1 Average age and age range of gross motor developmental milestones.

The earlier motor development stages—sitting, standing, and sometimes, crawling—are important for the development of walking. Developmental stages build on each other. Early milestones in most cases are prerequisites to later ones, with crawling being the exception as not all children crawl.[37]

Milestones are an important reference when a child appears to be late in development compared with typically developing children. For example, one of the hallmarks of CP is that the child may be late in achieving gross motor developmental milestones. In fact, that may be what first alerts parents or professionals to a problem.

However, being late in achieving milestones does not mean that a child will never achieve them or that the child cannot progress.

The development of function is under the control of the nervous system and is affected to varying degrees in CP. Function may improve somewhat without treatment, but treatment is essential to maximize function as early as possible, which is why early intervention is so important.

Measuring function

A number of standardized measurement (assessment) tools may be used to measure function. Examples include:

- DAYC (Developmental Assessment of Young Children) for infants and children from birth to five years
- Peabody Developmental Motor Scales for infants and children from birth to five years
- Bayley Scales of Infant and Toddler Development for infants and children from 1 to 42 months
- Gross Motor Function Measure (GMFM) for children with CP age five months to 16 years.

Information on these and other measurement tools is included in Appendix 1 (online).

As a parent, I never thought too much about walking. My two older children walked before their first birthdays and developed running and jumping skills without my ever having to notice or think about them. It is only when there is a problem that we begin to think about what walking actually involves.

Classification based on predominant motor type and topography

Order and simplification are the first steps toward the mastery of a subject—the actual enemy is the unknown.

Thomas Mann

Over the years, there has been much discussion of the classification of CP. Classification, or dividing into groups, is useful because it provides information about the nature of the condition and its severity (its level or magnitude). It also allows us to learn from people who have the condition at a similar level.

This section addresses classification of CP based on predominant motor type and topography. ("Predominant motor type" means the predominant abnormal muscle tone* and movement impairment, and "topography" means area of the body affected.) It also covers location of the brain injury and prevalence of CP by subtype. The next section looks at classification of CP based on functional ability.

---

* The resting tension in a person's muscles. A range of normal muscle tone exists. Tone is considered abnormal when it falls outside the range of normal or typical. It can be too low (hypotonia) or too high (hypertonia).

CP subtype based on predominant motor type

There are several subtypes of CP based on the predominant motor type. These include:

- Spasticity—spastic CP
- Dyskinesia—dyskinetic CP
- Ataxia—ataxic CP
- Hypotonia—hypotonic CP[4]

See Table 1.6.1.

Table 1.6.1 CP subtypes based on predominant motor type

CP SUBTYPE	EXPLANATION
Spasticity—spastic CP	Spasticity is a condition in which there is an abnormal increase in muscle tone or stiffness of muscle that can interfere with movement and speech, and be associated with discomfort or pain.[22]
Dyskinesia—dyskinetic CP	Dyskinesia is a condition in which there are "abnormal patterns of posture and/or movement associated with involuntary, uncontrolled, recurring, occasionally stereotyped movement patterns."[8] ("Stereotyped movement patterns" means the movements are in a particular pattern, specific to that person, which is repeated.) Dyskinetic CP can be subdivided into either dystonic or choreo-athetotic CP.[38] - **Dystonic (dystonia):** Dystonia is characterized by involuntary (unintended) muscle contractions that cause slow repetitive movements or abnormal postures that can sometimes be painful.[39] - **Choreo-athetotic (choreo-athetosis):** 　○ Chorea is characterized by jerky, dance-like movements.[3] 　○ Athetosis is characterized by slow, writhing movements.[3]

Cont'd.

CP SUBTYPE	EXPLANATION
Ataxia—ataxic CP	Ataxia means "without coordination." People with ataxic CP "experience a failure of muscle control in their arms and legs, resulting in a lack of balance and coordination or a disturbance of gait."[40]
Hypotonia—hypotonic CP	Hypotonia is a condition in which there is an abnormal decrease in muscle tone.[22] The muscles are floppy.

It is worth noting that these abnormal muscle tone or movement impairments may be present in other conditions, not just CP.

CP subtype based on topography

There are two methods of classifying CP subtypes based on topography. One is older (historical), and one has been more recently adopted (SCPE).

With the first method, the names of all the subtypes have the suffix "plegia," which is derived from the Greek word for stroke, although there are causes of CP other than a stroke. The prefixes in the names of the subtypes—"mono," "hemi," "di," "tri," and "quad," also derived from Greek, or Latin—indicate how many limbs are affected (see Table 1.6.2).*

---

* Occasionally, the terms "hemiparesis" for spastic hemiplegia, "diparesis" for spastic diplegia, and "quadriparesis" for spastic quadriplegia are used.[41]

Table 1.6.2 CP subtypes based on topography—historical

CP SUBTYPE	AREA OF BODY AFFECTED	
Monoplegia		Mono = One. One limb, usually one of the lower limbs.
Hemiplegia		Hemi = Half. Upper and lower limbs on one side of the body. The upper limb is usually more affected than the lower limb.
Diplegia		Di = Two. All limbs, but the lower limbs much more than the upper ones, which frequently show only fine motor impairment.
Triplegia		Tri = Three. Three limbs, usually the two lower limbs and one upper limb. The lower limb on the side of the upper limb involvement is usually more affected.
Quadriplegia		Quad = Four. All four limbs and the trunk; also known as tetraplegia.

One of the disadvantages of the historical classification system is a lack of precision.[8] However, this system has been and continues to be used extensively, particularly in the US.

The Surveillance of Cerebral Palsy in Europe network (SCPE) has developed a simpler classification method, also based on topography.[38] This method is now generally used in Europe and Australia. It identifies two main subtypes of CP: unilateral and bilateral (see Table 1.6.3).

Table 1.6.3 CP subtypes based on topography—SCPE

CP SUBTYPE	AREA OF BODY AFFECTED
Unilateral	One side of the body.
Bilateral	Both sides of the body.

Location of brain injury

Different subtypes of CP result from injury to different parts of the brain:

- Spasticity is associated with injury to the cerebrum.
- Dyskinesia is associated with injury to the basal ganglia and thalamus.
- Ataxia is associated with injury to the cerebellum.
- Hypotonia is associated with injury to the cerebrum and cerebellum.

Figure 1.6.1 summarizes CP subtypes, predominant motor types, topography, and location of brain injury.

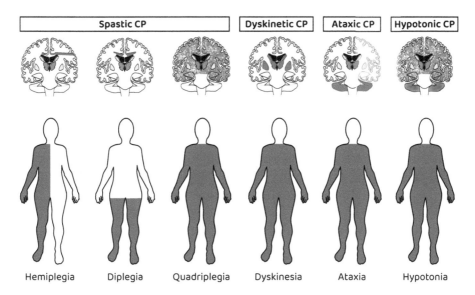

Figure 1.6.1 CP subtypes and location of brain injury (orange) and area of body affected (green).

Figure 1.6.1 shows:

- The extent of body involvement (green): regional involvement as in spastic hemiplegia and spastic diplegia; total body involvement as in spastic quadriplegia and the nonspastic forms of CP (i.e., dyskinesia, ataxia, and hypotonia).
- The location of the brain injury (orange) and CP subtype:
  - Injury primarily to the left cerebrum causing right side spastic hemiplegia (and vice versa)
  - Injury to both left and right cerebrum causing spastic diplegia
  - More extensive injury to both left and right cerebrum causing spastic quadriplegia
  - Injury to the basal ganglia and thalamus causing dyskinesia
  - Injury to the cerebellum causing ataxia
  - Injury to both left and right cerebrum and cerebellum causing hypotonia

Note that this is a *very* simplified explanation. In reality, CP is much more nuanced. For example, there may be more than one area of brain injury. In addition, particularly with a preterm birth, brain injury may happen more than once. As well, the brain injury can vary from very mild to very severe.

Knowledge of the brain injury sometimes confirms the symptoms seen in a child. MRI scans are becoming more routine with CP. However, up to 17 percent of children with CP have normal MRI brain scans.[3]

Recall that the brain injury in CP is unchanging (i.e., the size and location do not change), but "unchanging" may be a bit misleading since with time, growth, and maturation of the brain and other structures, the effects of the brain injury become more apparent in the form of motor delays and problems with other body systems.

Prevalence of CP by subtype

Figure 1.6.2 shows the prevalence of CP by predominant motor type and topography for almost 11,000 Australian children with CP.[4,42] While precise percentages of prevalence are different in other countries, the data in Figure 1.6.2 is from a large dataset and is consistent with studies from other countries.[43-46] It shows that:

- The predominant motor type is spastic (78 percent).
- Hemiplegia, diplegia, and quadriplegia each represent approximately one-third of the total.

Note that only spastic CP is subdivided by topography because the other subtypes (i.e., dyskinetic, ataxic, and hypotonic CP) generally affect the whole body.

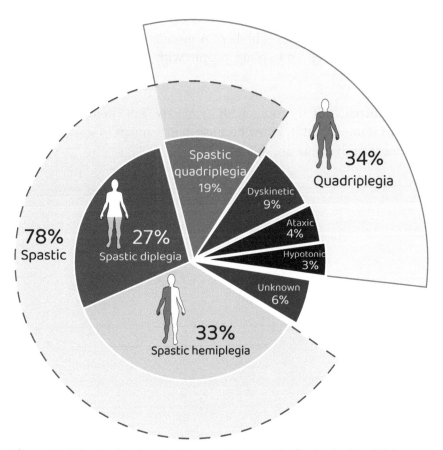

Figure 1.6.2 Predominant motor type and topography for Australian children with CP.[4,42]

It is important to note that different CP registers regard hypotonia differently. The Australian CP register includes hypotonia as a subtype of CP; the European CP register does not. Figure 1.6.2 shows that 3 percent of Australian children with CP were classified as having hypotonic CP.[4] One study found that only 46 percent of physicians who diagnose CP in the US and Canada would diagnose it in the case of hypotonia.[47] A diagnosis of CP is important because it may affect access to rehabilitation services in some countries.

Finally, it's important to understand that while CP is classified based on the predominant motor type, many individuals have secondary or co-occurring motor types. Data from the Australian CP register, for example, showed that 12 percent of individuals with spastic diplegia have co-occurring dyskinesia, and it is believed that the true prevalence of co-occurring motor types is higher.[4] A more recent report found that 50 percent of children and young people with CP had spasticity *and* dystonia.[48]

The co-occurrence of dystonia with spasticity has been underrecognized. This is important to know because management of spasticity and management of dystonia are different.

Classification based on functional ability

It is our choices, Harry, that show what we truly are,
far more than our abilities.

J.K. Rowling

A series of functional ability classification systems has been developed, with each having the same structure and common language. These systems include classifying CP based on:

- Functional mobility (as in movement from place to place)
- Manual ability (ability to handle objects)
- Communication ability
- Eating and drinking ability
- Visual function

Functional mobility

The Gross Motor Function Classification System (GMFCS) is a five-level classification system that describes the functional mobility of children and adolescents with CP.[49] The GMFCS and the expanded, revised version—GMFCS E&R[50]—includes descriptions for five age groups:

- 0 to 2 years
- 2 to 4 years
- 4 to 6 years
- 6 to 12 years
- 12 to 18 years

The emphasis is on the child's or adolescent's usual performance in their daily environment (i.e., their home and community).* By choosing which description best matches the child at their current age, they can be assigned a GMFCS level.

Table 1.7.1 describes the five levels. The severity of the movement limitations increases with each level, with level I having the fewest movement limitations and level V having the most. It is important to note, however, that the differences between the levels are not equal.

Table 1.7.1 Functional mobility across the five levels of the GMFCS[49,50]

GMFCS LEVEL	FUNCTIONAL MOBILITY
I	Walks without limitations
II	Walks with limitations
III	Walks using a handheld mobility device (assistive walking device)*
IV	Self-mobility with limitations; may use powered mobility†
V	Transported in a manual wheelchair

* Handheld mobility device (assistive walking device) includes canes, crutches, and walkers that do not support the weight of the trunk during walking.

† Powered mobility includes wheelchairs and scooters controlled by a joystick or electrical switch.

---

* In this context, "community" may be interpreted as "away from home." Moving about at home is generally easier since it is likely well suited or adapted to the person's needs. The community may be more challenging. It is important to keep in mind the impact of environmental and personal factors on what children and adolescents are able to do in their daily environment (home or community). See section 1.8, The International Classification of Functioning, Disability and Health.

The GMFCS levels are based on the method of functional mobility that best describes the child's performance after age six, but a child can be classified much earlier using these descriptions. They are relatively stable after age two.[49,51,52] In fact, stability into young adulthood has been demonstrated. McCormick and colleagues found that a GMFCS level observed around age 12 was highly predictive of motor function in early adulthood.[53]

Knowing a child's level offers insight into what the future may hold in terms of their mobility. It helps answer some of the many questions parents may have in the early days, such as, "Will my child walk?" or, "How serious is their CP?"

The full version of the GMFCS E&R is a short document and is included in **Useful web resources**. It contains further detail on functional mobility for each age and GMFCS level. It also includes a summary of the distinctions between each level to help determine which level most closely resembles a particular child's or adolescent's functional mobility. Useful illustrations have been developed based on the GMFCS for the two upper age bands (6 to 12 years and 12 to 18 years) by staff at the Royal Children's Hospital in Melbourne (see Figures 1.7.1 and 1.7.2).

GMFCS E & R between 6th and 12th birthday: Descriptors and illustrations

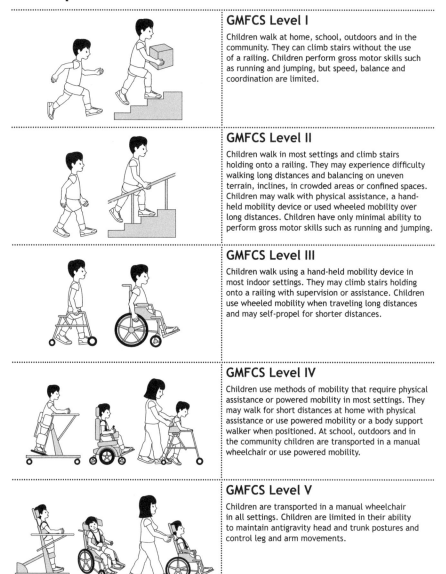

GMFCS Level I

Children walk at home, school, outdoors and in the community. They can climb stairs without the use of a railing. Children perform gross motor skills such as running and jumping, but speed, balance and coordination are limited.

GMFCS Level II

Children walk in most settings and climb stairs holding onto a railing. They may experience difficulty walking long distances and balancing on uneven terrain, inclines, in crowded areas or confined spaces. Children may walk with physical assistance, a hand-held mobility device or used wheeled mobility over long distances. Children have only minimal ability to perform gross motor skills such as running and jumping.

GMFCS Level III

Children walk using a hand-held mobility device in most indoor settings. They may climb stairs holding onto a railing with supervision or assistance. Children use wheeled mobility when traveling long distances and may self-propel for shorter distances.

GMFCS Level IV

Children use methods of mobility that require physical assistance or powered mobility in most settings. They may walk for short distances at home with physical assistance or use powered mobility or a body support walker when positioned. At school, outdoors and in the community children are transported in a manual wheelchair or use powered mobility.

GMFCS Level V

Children are transported in a manual wheelchair in all settings. Children are limited in their ability to maintain antigravity head and trunk postures and control leg and arm movements.

GMFCS descriptors: Palisano et al. (1997) Dev Med Child Neurol 39:214-23
CanChild: www.canchild.ca

Illustrations Version 2 © Bill Reid, Kate Willoughby, Adrienne Harvey and Kerr Graham, The Royal Children's Hospital Melbourne ERC151050

Figure 1.7.1 GMFCS E&R between 6th and 12th birthday: Descriptors and illustrations. Reproduced with kind permission from K. Graham and K. Willoughby, Royal Children's Hospital Melbourne, Australia.

GMFCS E & R between 12th and 18th birthday: Descriptors and illustrations

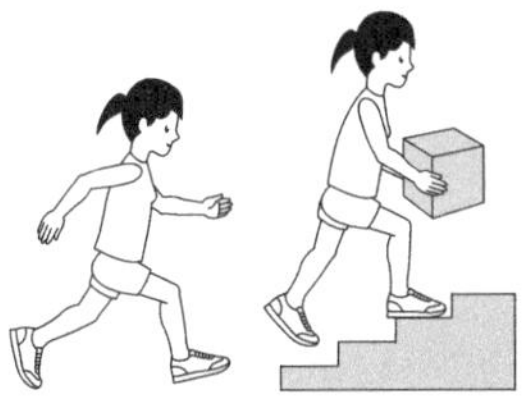

GMFCS Level I

Youth walk at home, school, outdoors and in the community. Youth are able to climb curbs and stairs without physical assistance or a railing. They perform gross motor skills such as running and jumping but speed, balance and coordination are limited.

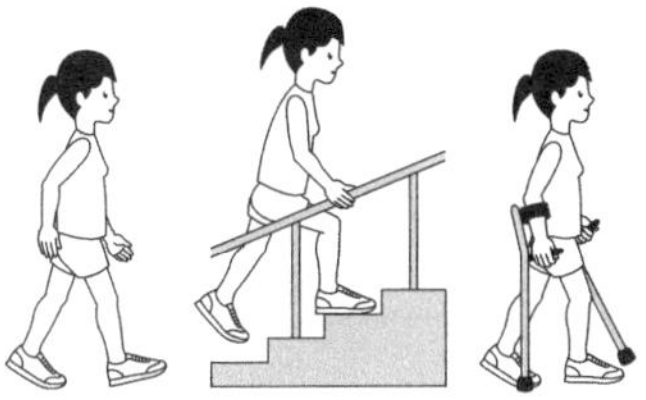

GMFCS Level II

Youth walk in most settings but environmental factors and personal choice influence mobility choices. At school or work they may require a hand held mobility device for safety and climb stairs holding onto a railing. Outdoors and in the community youth may use wheeled mobility when traveling long distances.

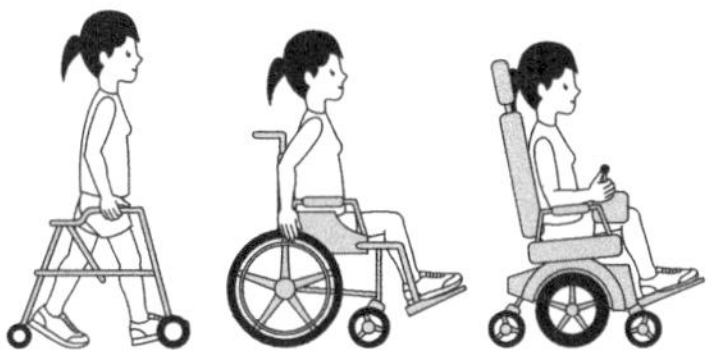

GMFCS Level III

Youth are capable of walking using a hand-held mobility device. Youth may climb stairs holding onto a railing with supervision or assistance. At school they may self-propel a manual wheelchair or use powered mobility. Outdoors and in the community youth are transported in a wheelchair or use powered mobility.

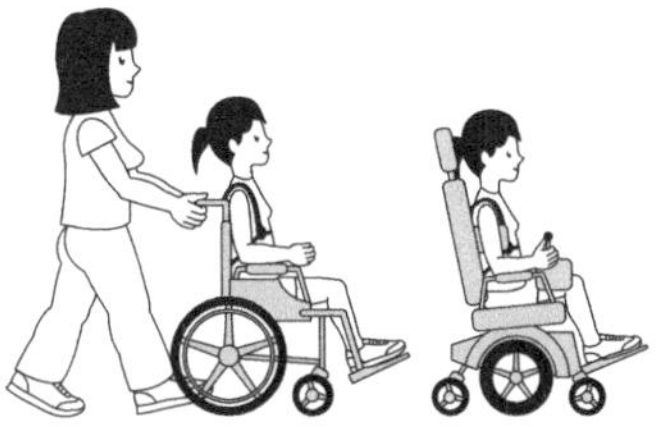

GMFCS Level IV

Youth use wheeled mobility in most settings. Physical assistance of 1-2 people is required for transfers. Indoors, youth may walk short distances with physical assistance, use wheeled mobility or a body support walker when positioned. They may operate a powered chair, otherwise are transported in a manual wheelchair.

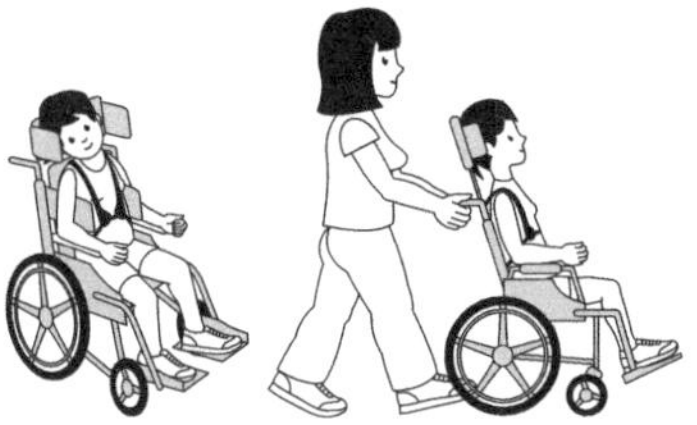

GMFCS Level V

Youth are transported in a manual wheelchair in all settings. Youth are limited in their ability to maintain antigravity head and trunk postures and control leg and arm movements. Self-mobility is severely limited, even with the use of assistive technology.

GMFCS descriptors: Palisano et al. (1997) Dev Med Child Neurol 39:214-23
CanChild: www.canchild.ca

Illustrations Version 2 © Bill Reid, Kate Willoughby, Adrienne Harvey and Kerr Graham, The Royal Children's Hospital Melbourne   ERC151050

Figure 1.7.2 GMFCS E&R between 12th and 18th birthday: Descriptors and illustrations. Reproduced with kind permission from K. Graham and K. Willoughby, Royal Children's Hospital Melbourne, Australia.

One use of the GMFCS has been classifying walking ability into three levels:[54]

- **Mild:** independent walker; GMFCS levels I–II
- **Moderate:** walker with aid; GMFCS level III
- **Severe:** wheelchair; GMFCS levels IV–V

In addition, the GMFCS led to the development of the gross motor development curves.[55,56] The curves show the change in gross motor function over time as measured by the Gross Motor Function Measure-66 (GMFM-66).[*] There are five curves, one for each GMFCS level (see Figure 1.7.3).

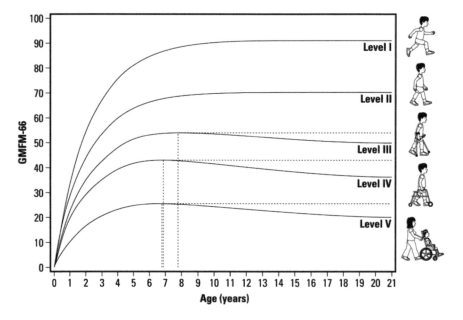

Figure 1.7.3 Gross motor curves in children with CP and the five levels of the GMFCS. Adapted with kind permission from *Cerebral Palsy: Science and Clinical Practice,* edited by B. Dan et al. (2014). Mac Keith Press.

The curves allow us to see how a child's gross motor function is likely to develop over time, as measured by the GMFM-66. The figure shows

---

[*] A standardized assessment tool used to evaluate the gross motor function of individuals with CP. It consists of 66 items that assess a wide range of gross motor skills. Also used is GMFM-88, which assesses 88 items. Each addresses five areas of increasing gross motor function: 1) lying and rolling, 2) sitting, 3) crawling and kneeling, 4) standing, and 5) walking, running, and jumping.

the average GMFM-66 score (vertical y-axis) at each GMFCS level by age (horizontal x-axis). Specifically, it shows:

- For each level there is an initial rapid rise in score to a peak, then it plateaus (levels I–II) or decreases (levels III–V).
- The score is highest for level I and lowest for level V.
- The dotted lines show the age at which the score peaks and the decrease from the peak to age 21 years for levels III–V (the oldest participants in the study were 21, so the shape of the curves after 21 are not known).
- Even a child at level I does not reach 100, the maximum, on the scale.

These curves are based on averages, and it is important to remember that some children were above and some below the line at each level.[55] Still, they are very useful. Why? Because they help answer some of the many questions parents have in the early days. Knowing a child's GMFCS level at age two, for example, allows parents to see how the child's gross motor function, as measured by the GMFM-66, is likely to develop over time. However, it is worth noting that the curves are not accurate before the age of two.

While remaining very realistic in expectations, the focus should be on helping the child reach their maximum possible gross motor function, not just hitting the average. The curves should guide, but not limit, a child's potential.

Tommy was born in 1994. The first GMFCS to age 12 was published in 1997, and the curves were published in 2002. Looking back, I can see how useful they could have been earlier in Tommy's life. Before these tools emerged, questions like, "Will our child walk?" were difficult for professionals to answer; they likely did not want to overpromise.

When I asked whether Tommy would walk, I was told he would walk before age seven but would likely need to use a wheelchair in college. As it turned out, Tommy began to walk independently just after his third birthday and continued to walk independently right through college. (In fact, my favorite photograph from his college graduation is one I took of the family and a friend walking to dinner that evening. It was special because not only was Tommy graduating, he was also walking unaided beside his dad and brothers. I sent a copy of that photograph, with great gratitude, to the many professionals who had treated him over the years.)

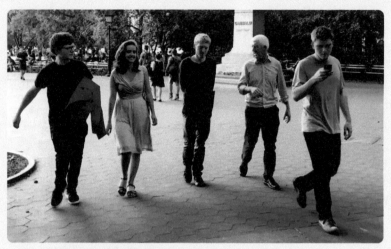

Tommy (far left), with a friend and his dad and brothers.

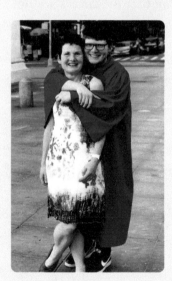

Tommy and me.

I do not have a record of Tommy's earlier GMFM-66 scores, but just before his 10th birthday his GMFM-66 score was 78. Plotting that score on the curves put him between levels I and II, and at that time he was classed as level II (walks with limitations). This accurately describes how Tommy walks today.

Manual ability

The Manual Ability Classification System (MACS) is a five-level classification system that describes how children and adolescents with CP age 4 to 18 years handle objects in daily activities.[57] The levels are based on the individual's ability to handle objects (relevant and age appropriate) and their need for assistance or adaptation. A separate Mini-MACS is available for children age one to four.[58]

Table 1.7.2 describes the five levels. Limitations of manual ability increase with increasing MACS level. As with the GMFCS, the differences between levels are not equal. The scale is used to classify overall ability to handle objects, *not* each hand separately. The emphasis is on the child's or adolescent's overall usual performance in their daily environment (their home, school, and community), rather than what is known to be their best performance.

Table 1.7.2 Ability to handle objects across the five levels of the MACS[57]

MACS LEVEL	ABILITY TO HANDLE OBJECTS
I	Handles objects easily and successfully
II	Handles most objects but with somewhat reduced quality and/or speed of achievement
III	Handles objects with difficulty; needs help to prepare and/or modify activities
IV	Handles a limited selection of easily managed objects in adapted situations
V	Does not handle objects and has severely limited ability to perform even simple actions

The full versions of the MACS and Mini-MACS are short documents and are included in **Useful web resources**. They provide further detail on each level and a summary of the distinctions between adjacent levels to help determine the most appropriate level for the individual.

An alternative to the MACS is the Bimanual Fine Motor Function (BFMF)[59,60,61] (see Figure 1.7.4). Unlike the MACS (and Mini-MACS), the BFMF assesses the child's ability to grasp, hold, and manipulate objects in *each* hand separately.[60] More information on the BFMF is included in **Useful web resources.**

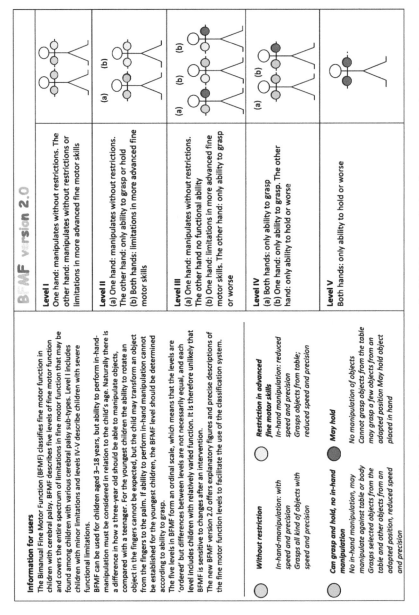

Figure 1.7.4 BFMF level identification chart. Reproduced with kind permission from Dr. Kate Himmelmann and Dr. Ann-Kristin Elvrum.

Communication ability

The Communication Function Classification System (CFCS) is a five-level classification system that describes everyday communication performance for children with CP.[62] Table 1.7.3 describes the five levels. Hidecker and colleagues have defined some key concepts used in this classification system:

> Communication occurs when a **sender** transmits a message, **and a receiver** understands the message ... **Unfamiliar conversational partners** are strangers or acquaintances who only occasionally communicate with the person. **Familiar conversational partners** such as relatives, caregivers, and friends may be able to communicate more effectively with the person because of previous knowledge and personal experiences ... All methods of communication performance are considered ... These include speech, gestures, behaviors, eye gaze, facial expressions, and augmentative and alternative communication (AAC).[62]

Table 1.7.3 Communication ability across the five levels of the CFCS[62]

CFCS LEVEL	COMMUNICATION ABILITY
I	Effective sender and receiver with unfamiliar and familiar partners
II	Effective but slower-paced sender and/or receiver with unfamiliar and/or familiar partners
III	Effective sender and receiver with familiar partners
IV	Inconsistent sender and/or receiver with familiar partners
V	Seldom-effective sender and receiver even with familiar partners

An alternative to the CFCS is the Viking Speech Scale (VSS),[63,64,65] but it addresses just speech. It is a four-point scale, with level I having the fewest limitations and level IV the most (see Table 1.7.4).

Table 1.7.4 Viking Speech Scale

VSS LEVEL	SPEECH UNDERSTANDABILITY
I	Speech is not affected by motor disorder.
II	Speech is imprecise but usually understandable to unfamiliar listeners.
III	Speech is unclear and not usually understandable to unfamiliar listeners out of context.
IV	No understandable speech.

More information on both the CFCS and VSS is included in **Useful web resources.**

Eating and drinking ability

The Eating and Drinking Ability Classification System (EDACS) is used for individuals with CP who are age three and older.[66] The EDACS assesses eating and drinking from two perspectives across the five levels:[66]

- **Safety:** For example, aspiration (food or liquid entering the airway or lungs instead of the esophagus) and choking (blockage of the airway by food)
- **Efficiency:** Amount of food and liquid lost from the mouth and time taken to eat

Table 1.7.5 describes the five levels.

Table 1.7.5 Eating and drinking ability across the five levels of the EDACS[66]

EDACS LEVEL	EATING AND DRINKING ABILITY
I	Eats and drinks safely and efficiently
II	Eats and drinks safely but with some limitations to efficiency
III	Eats and drinks with some limitations to safety; there may be limitations to efficiency
IV	Eats and drinks with significant limitations to safety
V	Unable to eat and drink safely—tube-feeding may be considered to provide nutrition

Useful illustrations for the EDACS from age three years have been developed focusing on the safety and efficiency aspects of feeding (see Figure 1.7.5).

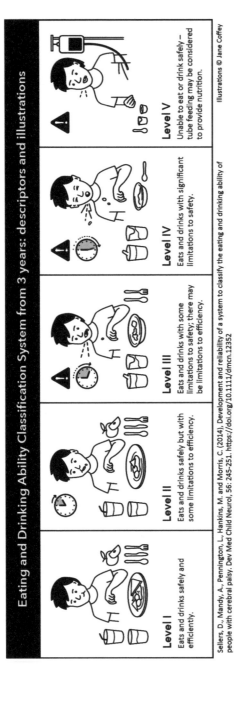

Eating and Drinking Ability Classification System from 3 years: descriptors and illustrations

Level I
Eats and drinks safely and efficiently.

Level II
Eats and drinks safely but with some limitations to efficiency.

Level III
Eats and drinks with some limitations to safety; there may be limitations to efficiency.

Level IV
Eats and drinks with significant limitations to safety.

Level V
Unable to eat or drink safely – tube feeding may be considered to provide nutrition.

Illustrations © Jane Coffey

Sellers, D., Mandy, A., Pennington, L., Hankins, M. and Morris, C. (2014), Development and reliability of a system to classify the eating and drinking ability of people with cerebral palsy. Dev Med Child Neurol, 56: 245-251. https://doi.org/10.1111/dmcn.12352

Figure 1.7.5 EDACS from three years of age. Reproduced with kind permission from Dr. Diane Sellers; © Jane Coffey.

A Mini-EDACS has been developed for children with CP from age 18 to 36 months.[67] More information on the EDACS and Mini-EDACS is included in **Useful web resources.**

Visual function

The Visual Function Classification System (VFCS) is for individuals with CP from the age of one. Table 1.7.6 describes the five levels.

Table 1.7.6 Visual function across the five levels of the VFCS[68]

VFCS LEVEL	VISUAL FUNCTION
I	Uses visual function easily and successfully in vision-related activities
II	Uses visual function successfully but needs self-initiated compensatory strategies
III	Uses visual function but needs some adaptations
IV	Uses visual function in very adapted environments but performs just part of vision-related activities
V	Does not use visual function even in very adapted environments

More information on the VFCS is included in **Useful web resources.**

Using classification systems

Together, the various classification systems provide a lot of information, and each is valid and reliable.[*,68,69] Because families can understand (and assign) classification system levels,[69,70] the systems can help with communication between medical professionals and families. They also help with good planning of care both in the present and into the future since they are stable over time.[69] However, it is because they are stable over time that they should not and cannot be used to detect change after an intervention.[70] Robust research is one of the backbones for improving clinical care for individuals with CP. The classification systems are very useful for research since participants can be better identified for research studies.

Finally, although CP is a single diagnosis, it is far from a uniform condition. Similar to autism, a name change, from "cerebral palsy" to "cerebral palsy spectrum disorder," has been suggested.[71]

---

* A good classification system must be:
  * **Valid:** It measures what it claims to measure.
  * **Reliable:** It provides the same answer when used by different people or by the same person at different times.
  * **Accurate:** It measures how close a value is to its true value (e.g., how close an arrow gets to the target).
  * **Precise:** It measures how repeatable a measurement is (e.g., how close the second arrow is to the first one, regardless of whether either is near the target).

These same principles also apply to measurement (assessment) tools. A kitchen scale (weighing scale) can be used to illustrate the different concepts:
  * If the scale claims to measure weight and does so, then the scale is valid.
  * If it provides the same reading regardless of who uses it or when they use it, then the scale is reliable.
  * If the reading is correct when a known standard weight is weighed, then the scale is accurate.
  * If repeated weighings of the same item give the same reading (whether accurate or not), then the scale is precise.

The International Classification of Functioning, Disability and Health

The individual is rarely going to be altered very much,
whereas the environment slowly but surely can.

Tom Shakespeare

The International Classification of Functioning, Disability and Health (ICF), a framework briefly addressed in the Introduction, is considered here in more detail and in the context of CP. The ICF was developed by WHO* in 2001 to help show the impact of a health condition at different levels and how those levels are interconnected. It tells us to look at the full picture—to look at the person with a disability in their life situation. The "F" in the short-form name of the framework (the ICF) stands for "functioning," which shows where its emphasis lies.

The framework provides a way of looking at the concepts of health and disability. It shows that every human being can experience a decrease in health and thereby experience some disability. That is, disability is

---

* When WHO (the World Health Organization) was established in 1948, it defined health as "... a state of complete physical, mental, and social well-being and not merely the absence of disease or infirmity." This interesting and broad definition has stood the test of time: it has never been amended.

not something that happens only to a minority of people. The ICF thus "mainstreams" disability and recognizes it as a widespread human experience. See Figure 1.8.1.

> You might wonder why we need a framework to understand a health condition. As I became familiar with the ICF, I could really see its usefulness. The idea that every human being can experience a decrease in health and therefore experience some disability is useful because it illustrates that people don't fit neatly into one of two boxes (metaphorically speaking): healthy or disabled. There is, rather, a continuum between health and disability. The framework is helpful because it focuses on how a person with CP functions in their life.

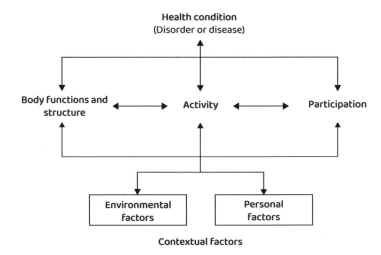

Figure 1.8.1 International Classification of Functioning, Disability and Health (ICF). Reproduced with kind permission from WHO.

The framework describes three levels of human functioning and disability as difficulty functioning at one or more of these three levels:[1]

- **Body functions and structure** refers to functioning at the level of the body or a body part.* For example, spasticity, muscle weakness,

---

* WHO formally defines "body functions" as physiological functions of body systems (including psychological functions). "Body structures" are defined as anatomical parts of the body such as organs, limbs, and their components.

pain, and cognition are at this level. Impairments are defined as problems in body functions and structure.

- **Activity** is performing a task or action by an individual; for example, walking or getting dressed. Activity limitations are difficulties an individual may have in performing activities.
- **Participation** is involvement in life situations. Playing sports with friends or attending school are examples. Participation restrictions are difficulties an individual may experience being involved in life situations.

The framework also includes factors that influence any of the three levels of functioning (termed "contextual factors"):

- **Environmental factors** make up the physical, social, and attitudinal environment in which people live. Examples include structural barriers at home and in the community, such as steps or stairs without handrails in the house, or a school with stairs but no elevator.
- **Personal factors** include gender, age, social background, education, past and present experiences, and other factors that influence how the person experiences disability. Examples include a person's attitude, determination, motivation, and resilience.

The three levels of human functioning, plus environmental and personal factors, are all interconnected with the health condition. The ICF shifts the focus from the *cause* to the *impact* of a health condition at the different levels.

Regarding activity, the ICF distinguishes between motor capacity and motor performance:

- **Motor capacity** is what a person can do in a standardized, controlled environment (e.g., a child at an appointment and walking on a smooth surface with the medical professional and parent watching and encouraging them).
- **Motor performance** is what a person actually does in their daily environment (e.g., a child walking in a crowded playground on uneven surfaces).

There is a third concept to keep in mind when considering activity: motor capability, which is what a person can do in their daily environment.[72]

For example, a child may be able to ride a bike to school—they have the capability—but they may choose not to. Their performance is influenced by their choice. Physical and social environment and personal factors such as motivation influence the relationship between capacity, capability, and performance.[72]

A series of "F-words" has been developed and inserted into the different areas of the ICF, providing a useful adaptation of the framework (see Figure 1.8.2).[73] "Fitness," "functioning," "friends," "family," "fun," and "future" are highlighted as areas of focus for the child with a health condition. Indeed, these also apply to adults. A number of useful videos on the F-words are included in **Useful web resources.**

I've observed how becoming familiar with the ICF has influenced my thinking over the years. In the early days, I was very focused on issues at the level of body functions and structure. Later I came to understand the relationship between the three levels. For example, orthopedic surgery leads to improvements at the level of body functions and structure addressing muscle and bone problems. As a result, the child may walk more easily and their walking might consume less energy. This is an improvement at the activity level. If walking is less tiring, the child might be able to keep up and do more with their peers—an improvement at the participation level. I also came to understand that treatments need to benefit a child at the level of activity and/or participation rather than purely at the level of body functions and structure. It is important to keep in mind that a treatment at one level will not necessarily help the child at another.

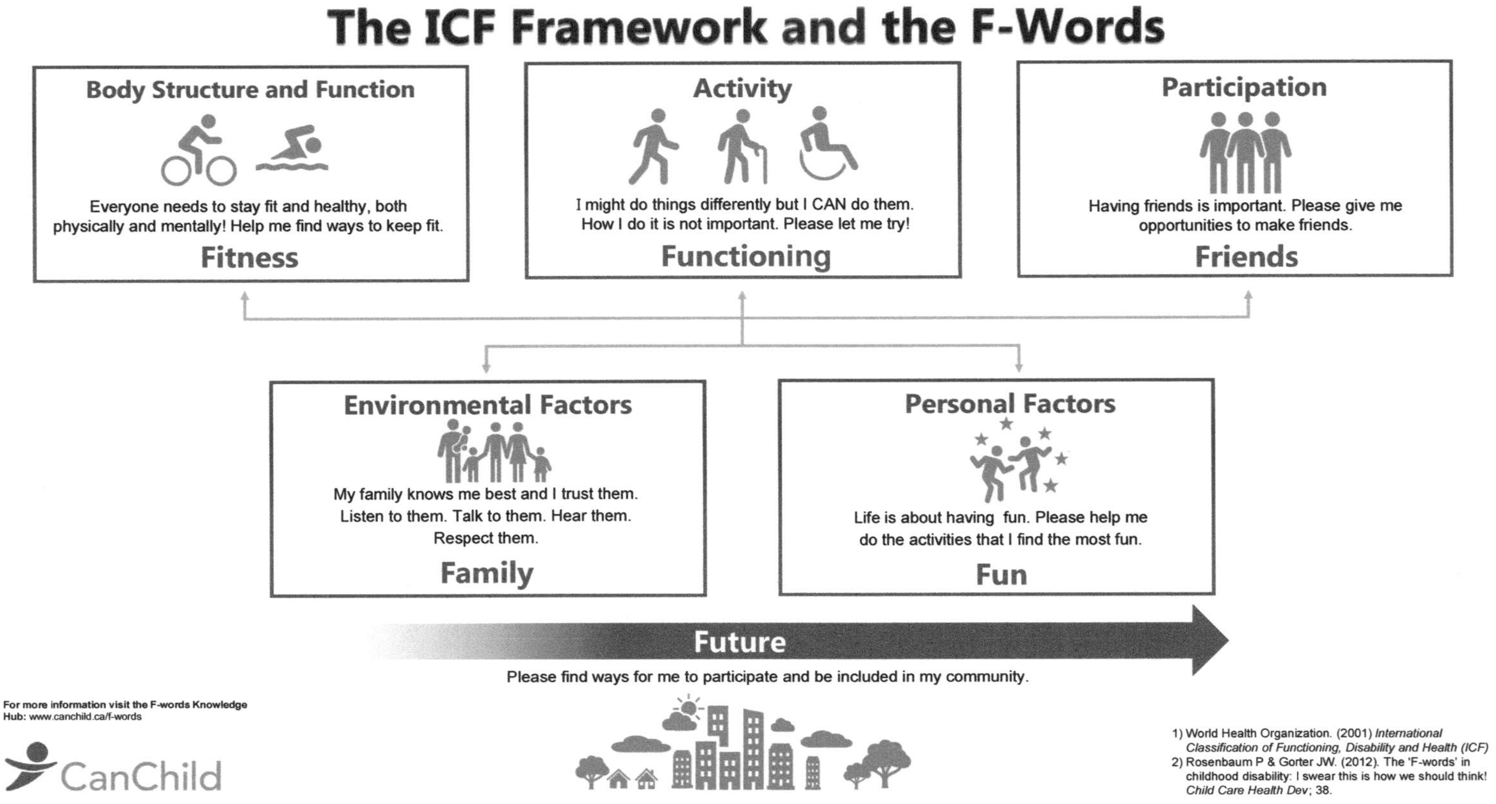

Figure 1.8.2 The ICF framework[1] and the F-words.[73] Reproduced with kind permission from CanChild.

Key points Chapter 1

- CP is a group of conditions caused by an injury to the developing brain that can result in a variety of motor and other problems that affect how the child functions. Because the injury occurs in a developing brain and growing child, problems often change over time, even though the brain injury itself is unchanging.
- CP is a lifelong condition. There is currently no cure, nor is one imminent, but good management and treatment can help alleviate some or many of the effects of the brain injury.
- Seventy to 80 percent of CP cases are associated with prenatal factors, and birth asphyxia (insufficient oxygen during birth) plays a relatively minor role.
- Infants who are born preterm (earlier than 37 weeks) or who have low birth weight have a higher risk of CP.
- The current CP birth prevalence for high-income countries is declining and is now 1.6 per 1,000 live births. It is higher for low- and middle-income countries.
- The most recent report from the Australian Cerebral Palsy Register shows a decrease in both prevalence and severity of CP.
- Using certain standardized tests in combination with clinical examination and medical history, a diagnosis of CP can often accurately be made before six months corrected age.
- Confirmation of the presence of a brain injury by magnetic resonance imaging (MRI) occurs in many but not all individuals with CP. Up to 17 percent of children given the diagnosis of CP have normal MRI brain scans.
- Early diagnosis is very important because it allows for early intervention. Early intervention helps to achieve better functional outcomes for the child.
- CP can be classified based on the predominant motor type (the predominant abnormal muscle tone and movement impairment) and topography (area of the body affected).
- A number of classification systems describe the functional mobility (as in movement from place to place), manual ability (ability to handle objects), communication ability, eating and drinking ability, and visual function of individuals with CP.

Spastic diplegia

Introduction

Nothing in life is to be feared, it is only to be understood. Now is the time to understand more, so that we may fear less.

Marie Curie

The title of this book is *Spastic Diplegia—Bilateral Cerebral Palsy*. "Spastic diplegia" is the term historically used to describe this condition, and it remains in use today in the US. The term "spastic diplegia" derives from "spastic" (the type of high tone), "di" (meaning two, referring to the two affected lower limbs), and "plegia" (the Greek word for stroke). Over the past 20 years, the term "bilateral spastic CP," or simply "bilateral CP," has been adopted in Europe and Australia because it is thought to provide a more accurate description of the condition. "Bilateral" refers to two sides of the body being affected. The three terms "spastic diplegia," "bilateral spastic CP," and "bilateral CP" are all used in the scientific literature. In this book, written in the US, we use the term "spastic diplegia."

With spastic diplegia, the lower limbs are much more affected than the upper limbs, which frequently show only fine motor impairment.

Spasticity is the most common type of atypical tone present, although dystonia can be present as well.

As noted in Chapter 1, the Gross Motor Function Classification System (GMFCS) offers an indication of the severity of the condition. This book is relevant to those at GMFCS levels I, II, and III: those who are capable of walking independently or with an assistive walking device. GMFCS levels I, II, and III account for the majority of individuals with spastic diplegia.

This chapter explains spastic diplegia from birth through adolescence. It should contribute to your understanding of how the condition arises and develops over time. It provides information intended to help parents understand the diagnosis and what to anticipate as their child grows to adulthood. It provides adolescents and adults with an understanding of their condition. Chapter 3 addresses the management of the condition during childhood and adolescence. Chapter 4 is devoted to spastic diplegia in adulthood.

Physical features

Gage, an orthopedic surgeon, described the motor problems of spastic diplegia as follows:[74]

> *The involvement is primarily in the lower extremities with relatively normal upper extremity function … Most … children will walk, although balance, particularly posterior balance, is a … problem. The "typical" gait of a child with diplegia … is one of flexion, adduction, and internal rotation at the hips and flexion at the knees. The feet usually have a valgus hindfoot and … abducted forefoot.*[74]

In their 2007 book, Horstmann and Bleck, also both orthopedic surgeons, described it as follows:[75]

> *When we observe the posture and gait of a child with spastic diplegia anywhere in the world it is as though each child came from the same mold. The common pattern … is flexed, adducted, and internally rotated hips … We see an increased anterior*

pelvic tilt, lumbar lordosis, either flexed or hyperextended knees, and equinus.

Table 2.1.1 explains and illustrates the typical physical features of spastic diplegia. Together, these features paint a picture of the movement and posture problems of spastic diplegia: of a child who walks on their toes with flexed (bent) knees and hips and whose bones are twisted.

Table 2.1.1 Typical physical features of spastic diplegia GMFCS levels I, II, and III

TERM USED IN DESCRIPTIONS	EXPLANATION	ILLUSTRATION
Lumbar lordosis	An exaggerated inward curve in the lumbar region of the spine, often called a swayback.	
Anterior pelvic tilt	A tipping forward of the pelvis to the front. (The triangle indicates the pelvis.)	
Adduction and internal rotation at the hips	Adduction is movement toward the middle of the body. Internal rotation is a twisting movement around the long axis of a bone toward the middle of the body. With adduction and internal rotation at the hips, the thigh turns inward and toward the middle of the body.	

Cont'd.

TERM USED IN DESCRIPTIONS	EXPLANATION	ILLUSTRATION
Flexion at the hips and knees	The hips and knees are bent.	
Hyperextended knees	"Hyperextended" means beyond straight or over-straightened. This is also termed "genu recurvatum." The knees on the left are hyperextended; the knees on the right are typical.	
Abducted forefoot	The front part of the foot (forefoot) moves away (outward) from the back part of the foot.	
Valgus hindfoot	The heels of both feet are turned away from the middle of the body to an atypical degree (i.e., the heels are turned outward). This is also termed "everted feet" or "eversion."	
Equinus	The toes are pointing downward (plantar flexed). In walking, this is referred to as toe walking or equinus gait.	

This chapter explains how an infant born with what appears to be typical bones, muscles, and joints can grow into a child who fits the descriptions above. I write "appears to be typical" because research is ongoing; there may be slight differences between the bones, muscles, and joints of an infant with spastic diplegia and those of a typically developing infant. Our understanding may change over time.

Distribution across classification systems

The effects of the brain injury can extend beyond movement and posture. Several classification systems for individuals with CP were introduced in section 1.7, including classification on the basis of:

- Functional mobility: Gross Motor Function Classification System (GMFCS)
- Ability to handle objects: Manual Ability Classification System (MACS)
- Communication ability: Communication Function Classification System (CFCS)
- Eating and drinking ability: Eating and Drinking Ability Classification System (EDACS)
- Visual function: Visual Function Classification System (VFCS)

Figure 2.1.1 summarizes the percentage distribution of children with spastic diplegia across the five levels of the GMFCS, MACS, CFCS, and of children with bilateral spastic CP* across the EADCS.[43-46,76-79] No data was found for the VFCS.

---

* Spastic diplegia and spastic quadriplegia; breakdown not available.

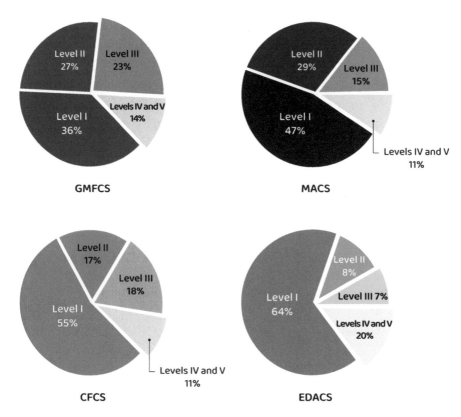

Figure 2.1.1 Distribution of children with spastic diplegia across the GMFCS, [43–46,76–78] MACS,[46,77] and CFCS[46] (top row and bottom left). Distribution of children with bilateral spastic CP across the EADCS[79] (bottom right).

Figure 2.1.1 shows that in the studies cited:

- Sixty-three percent of children with spastic diplegia were at levels I and II for GMFCS, while 76 percent were at levels I and II for MACS. This shows that the lower limbs are more affected than the upper limbs.
- Seventy-two percent of children with spastic diplegia were at levels I and II for CFCS.
- Seventy-two percent of children with bilateral spastic CP (i.e., both spastic diplegia and spastic quadriplegia) were at levels I and II for EDACS. It is expected that if those with spastic diplegia alone were considered, the percentage would be higher.

Furthermore, the level at which an individual functions on one of these classification systems can sometimes, though not always, be related to how they function on another.

Co-occurring motor type

With spastic diplegia, the predominant motor type is spasticity. However, individuals with spastic diplegia sometimes also have co-occurring, or secondary, motor types. Data from the Australian CP register shows that 12 percent of individuals with spastic diplegia (all GMFCS levels) have co-occurring dyskinesia, 2 percent have co-occurring ataxia, and 1 percent have co-occurring hypotonia.[*42] It is believed that the true prevalence of co-occurring motor types is higher[4] and the presence of dystonia with spasticity has been underrecognized.[48] A recent study found that 50 percent of children and young people with CP (all sub-types) had spasticity *and* dystonia.[48] This finding is important because the management of spasticity and dystonia is different.

Associated problems

A large Australian study reported on the prevalence of associated problems (i.e., problems with other body systems) among children aged five with spastic diplegia (all GMFCS levels).[80] See Figure 2.1.2.

---

* For those who acquired CP in the prenatal or perinatal period only.

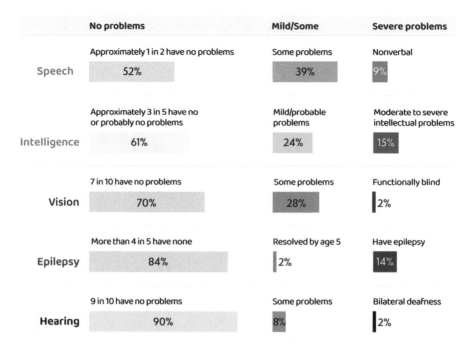

Figure 2.1.2 Prevalence of associated problems among children age five with spastic diplegia (all GMFCS levels).

Figure 2.1.2 shows that a proportion of children with spastic diplegia (all GMFCS levels) have problems in the areas of speech, intelligence (cognition), vision, epilepsy, and hearing of varying severity. Not shown in the figure is that more than 90 percent of children had none or only one severe associated problem.[80] As well, the prevalence and severity of associated problems were found to be greater in children at higher GMFCS levels compared with those at lower GMFCS levels.[80] Section 2.10 addresses associated problems in more detail.

Since spastic diplegia affects the lower limbs much more than the upper, this book focuses on the lower limbs and functional mobility for individuals with spastic diplegia.

Finally, where possible, we cite research studies relevant to those with spastic diplegia GMFCS levels I to III. Where studies include multiple subtypes, we aim to give an indication of the proportion of individuals with spastic diplegia and/or GMFCS level. Sometimes, data is available only for bilateral CP (not distinguishing diplegia and quadriplegia). We note this where included. Sometimes, we include information about CP in general, where this is deemed useful.

USEFUL WEB RESOURCES

Tommy had a CT scan when he was approximately one year old; phrases like "significant brain damage," "not much active brain," and "go home and mind the other children" conveyed the consultant's concern about what he saw on the scan. I was perplexed: how could this consultant say these things when he had never actually met our very alert and engaging child? It turned out Tommy has normal intelligence.

Those two descriptions of physical features by Drs. Gage, Horstmann, and Bleck described Tommy pretty accurately as a young child. In the early days, I thought the way Tommy walked was particular to him. Later, as I observed other people with spastic diplegia, I realized Tommy's manner of walking was characteristic of the condition. The concept that each child with spastic diplegia "came from the same mold" really resonated with me.

In hindsight, the only differences between Tommy and his two older brothers (who do not have spastic diplegia) as a baby were that he cried incessantly for the first three months, he was difficult to feed, and his legs felt strong and stiff from birth. That early stiffness was probably spasticity, though I would only become familiar with the term much later. The photograph below shows our eldest son holding a very rigid Tommy.

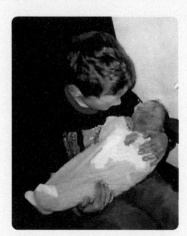

Tommy and his brother, Patrick.

The brain injury

The greater danger for most of us lies not in setting our aim too high and falling short; but in setting our aim too low, and achieving our mark.

Michelangelo

In terms of brain injuries, *when* and *where* (i.e., the timing in development and the location in the brain) an injury occurs determines the effects and severity of that injury, which translates to the subtype of CP.

Spastic diplegia is most commonly associated with preterm birth or an injury in the late second or early third trimester.[74,81] In this section, we briefly address the typical brain injury that causes spastic diplegia.

The classic brain injury of spastic diplegia is periventricular leukomalacia (PVL), explained as follows:

- **Periventricular:** "Peri" means around, "ventricular" means relating to the ventricles in the brain. The ventricles* are the black areas

---

* Interconnected fluid-filled cavities that produce, circulate, and contain cerebrospinal fluid, which protects the brain and spinal cord.

shown in Figure 2.2.1. The injury (orange area) occurs *near* these ventricles; hence the term "periventricular," which means around the ventricles.

• **Leukomalacia:** "Leuko" means white and "malacia" means abnormal softening of tissue. The term "leukomalacia," therefore, means softening of the white tissue.

The full term, "periventricular leukomalacia," describes the injury and means softening of the white tissue (white matter) around the ventricles.

Figure 2.2.1 shows the areas of the body that may be associated with the brain injury of spastic diplegia. The white matter in the area of injury includes the motor tracts (that control movement and posture, pink lines) and sensory tracts (that deliver sensory information, green lines) between the brain and spinal cord.

The tracts closest to the ventricles relate to the ankle, those next closest relate to the knee, and those next closest relate to the hip. We will see later that this mirrors the pattern of problems in spastic diplegia: the ankle is more involved than the knee, which in turn is more involved than the hip. There is less upper limb involvement in spastic diplegia, and as shown in the diagram, those tracts are even further from the site of the injury. The injury is usually bilateral (affecting both sides of the brain), but it can be uneven. The severity of spastic diplegia depends on the timing and the magnitude of the brain injury. The injury interrupts both motor and sensory communication. Thus, while movement is affected, other body systems may also be involved.

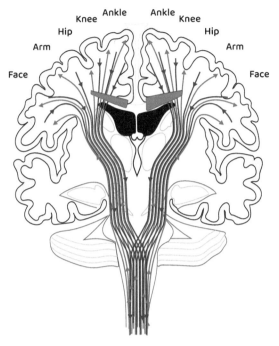

Knee Ankle Ankle Knee
Hip Hip
Arm Arm
Face Face

Figure 2.2.1 An example of brain injury resulting in spastic diplegia. The motor tracts (pink) descend from the cerebrum to the spinal cord, and the sensory tracts (green) ascend from the spinal cord to the cerebrum. The ventricles are the black areas. The orange area indicates the injury.

It is important to remember that this is a simplified explanation and, in reality, it is much more nuanced, unique to the individual, and complex. For example, there may be more than one area of brain injury. In addition, particularly with preterm birth, brain injury may happen more than once. The timing in development when the injury occurs is important because the areas of the brain that are developing at the time of the injury are the most vulnerable.

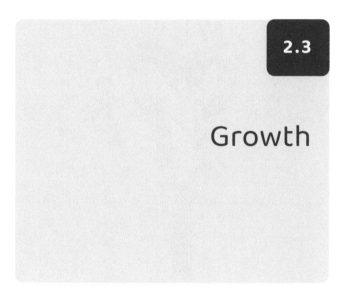

2.3

Growth

You have to do your own growing no
matter how tall your grandfather was.
Abraham Lincoln

The musculoskeletal problems in spastic diplegia develop in proportion to growth; therefore, an understanding of growth is helpful.

Growth occurs in three major phases during a child's life: birth to age three, three years to puberty, and puberty to maturity. Of the three phases, two are of *rapid* growth: from birth to three years and during puberty.[82] The rate of growth that occurs in these two phases is particularly important for the child with spastic diplegia because musculoskeletal problems emerge with growth.

It is worth noting that there are slight differences in growth between boys and girls with CP and typically developing peers. A large US study of growth in children and adolescents with CP led to the development of growth charts for boys and girls with CP age 2 to 20. These were developed for each GMFCS level.[83,84] The study found that children and adolescents with CP (all subtypes) are shorter than typically developing peers (see Figures 2.3.1 and 2.3.2). Similar trends in height difference among children and adolescents with CP have been observed in other parts of the world.[85]

These growth charts are included in **Useful web resources.**

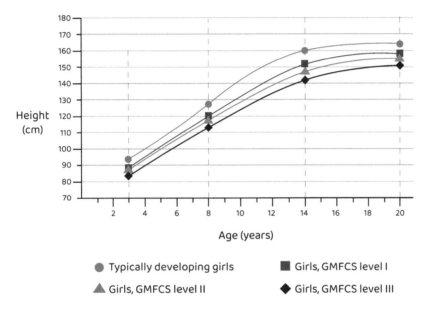

Figure 2.3.1 Height of girls with CP compared with typically developing peers. Data shows the 50th percentile height at various ages. Data collated and compiled from references.[83,84,86,87]

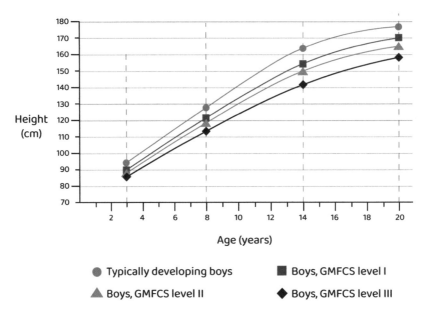

Height (cm) / Age (years)

- ● Typically developing boys
- ■ Boys, GMFCS level I
- ▲ Boys, GMFCS level II
- ◆ Boys, GMFCS level III

Figure 2.3.2 Height of boys with CP compared with typically developing peers. Data shows the 50th percentile height at various ages. Data collated and compiled from references.[83,84,88,89]

Since growth is such an important factor in spastic diplegia, I would advise parents to keep a growth chart for their child to stay focused on growth. I suggest you print the appropriate chart (boy or girl with CP and relevant GMFCS level) included in **Useful web links**.

Though any growth chart shows how much a typical child grows each year, an experienced parent knows that a child does not grow evenly throughout the year. Sometimes it felt like our sons shot up overnight. (I found this often followed a period of them eating more than usual.)

The difference in height between people with CP and typically developing peers was borne out at home: Tommy is not as tall as his two brothers.

The fact that the first three years are a period of very rapid growth is to some extent unfortunate as these years coincide with the time before diagnosis or when we parents are only just learning about and coming to terms with the diagnosis. This emphasizes the importance of early diagnosis so that needed early intervention can occur.

Bones, joints, muscles, and movements

It is not by muscle, speed, or physical dexterity that great things are achieved, but by reflection, force of character, and judgment.

Marcus Tullius Cicero

This section may seem like a physics and biology lesson, but because spastic diplegia affects the bones, joints, muscles, and movements, a basic understanding of them all helps enormously in understanding both the condition and its treatment.

Bones form the framework of the body, with the bones, joints, and muscles working together as levers to perform movement. In physics, a lever is a simple machine with four key components:

- A lever (a rigid bar)
- A fulcrum (a point about which the lever pivots)
- A resisting force (or load, such as a weight to be moved)
- An applied force (or effort; something that is doing the moving) (see Figure 2.4.1)

An example of a lever in humans is lifting a weight:

- The lower leg bones are the lever.
- The knee joint is the fulcrum.
- The object being lifted is the resisting force.
- The contraction of the knee extensor muscle creates the applied force.

Muscles provide the action; the bones just follow.

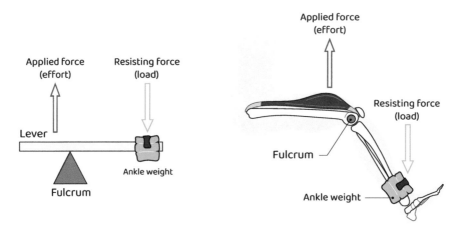

Figure 2.4.1 A lever (left) and the corresponding parts in the human leg (right).

Both the resisting force and applied force act on the lever at a distance from the fulcrum, which creates a torque or rotation (also called a "moment") about the fulcrum. This distance is called the force's "lever arm" (or "moment arm"). Even if the force stays constant, when the lever arm increases in length, the torque increases, and vice versa. Using the example in Figure 2.4.1, if the ankle weight were moved closer to the fulcrum (knee), effectively shortening the lever arm, a smaller applied force (i.e., muscle contraction) would be required to lift it.

As explained, muscles contract to produce force. The force produced can be very small (e.g., to pick up a feather) or very large (e.g., to pick up a kettlebell).

There are three types of muscles in the body:

- **Cardiac:** Muscle that forms the bulk of the wall of the heart
- **Smooth:** Muscle located in the walls of hollow internal structures such as the blood vessels, stomach, and intestines
- **Skeletal:** Muscle attached (mostly) to bones

Spastic diplegia primarily affects skeletal muscle.* Skeletal muscles contract to produce movement or maintain posture. The bones cannot stand up on their own; gravity would pull them down. When muscles contract, in addition to causing movement, they exert force, which keeps the body erect. Without these forces opposing gravity, the bones would collapse in a heap on the ground.

In a sense, the bones are like the limbs of a marionette (or puppet, see Figure 2.4.2). The marionette cannot stand up on its own.

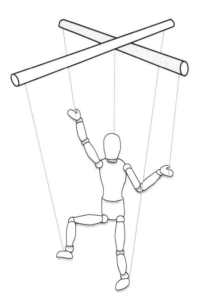

Figure 2.4.2 A marionette (puppet).

---

* There are some reports of smooth muscle being affected in CP.[90,91,92]

There are three types of muscle contractions:

- **Concentric (shortening):** For example, when going up a flight of stairs, the quadriceps (the muscles in front of the knee joint) contract concentrically—they shorten so that the knee extends.
- **Eccentric (lengthening):** For example, when going down a flight of stairs, the quadriceps (the same muscle that is involved in going up the stairs) contract eccentrically—they lengthen so that the knee bends. The lengthening contraction controls the bending of the knee against gravity.
- **Isometric (no change in length):** For example, when maintaining a posture (i.e., opposing the force of gravity), the muscles contract isometrically, without getting longer or shorter.

Every muscle has its own length when it is at rest. Muscles produce optimal force in the middle of that resting length.

While the details of the different types of contractions are not important in understanding spastic diplegia as such, it is helpful to keep in mind that during most movements (e.g., walking), muscles move in fractions of a second between these different types of contractions.

Muscles also contain noncontractile elements—that is, elements that are incapable of contracting. These form the tendon and various sheaths (enveloping or covering tissue). The tendon is the cord-like structure that attaches the muscle to the bone. The Achilles tendon, for example, attaches the gastrocnemius and soleus muscles—both calf muscles—to the heel. The combination of the muscle, tendon, and various sheaths is collectively known as the muscle-tendon unit (MTU).

Note also that there is a difference between muscle strength and muscle power: both are important for everyday activities like walking and running. Muscle strength is the amount of force that a muscle can generate during a specific movement—for example, the weight you can lift at the gym in a single repetition. Muscle power is the rate of force production (i.e., how fast the force is being produced). There is a strength aspect to power, but it is also about the speed of the movement. Jumping is an example of a power-based activity.

Something else to consider is range of motion (ROM), also called "range of movement," which is a measure of joint flexibility. The actual ROM through which a joint can be passively moved is measured in degrees. An instrument called a goniometer* is used to measure the ROM of a joint. (See Figure 2.4.3.) A video about measuring ROM is included in **Useful web resources.**

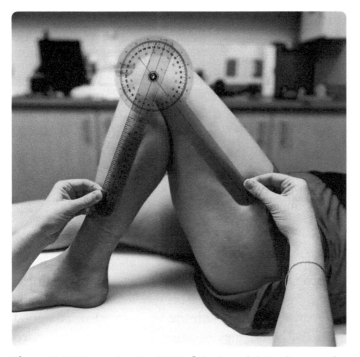

Figure 2.4.3 Measuring the ROM of the knee joint using a goniometer.

Table 2.4.1 explains the movements, joint ROMs, and key muscles for the lower limbs. This table is included as a reference and may be helpful at different times; for example, it may be useful to take it to some appointments. Below are some relevant points:

• Muscles are generally arranged in pairs around a joint. The muscles on one side of the joint move the joint in one direction, while the muscles on the other side of the joint move the joint in the opposite direction. Key muscles are identified at each joint, but minor muscles have not been included.

---

* A goniometer is like a movable protractor, used for measuring angles, as shown in Figure 2.4.3.

- Movements typically affected by spasticity are shown on the left side of the table and are indicated **with a green background**. *Some, but not necessarily all, of the muscles responsible for those movements may be affected by spasticity.* The table shows the movements typically affected by spasticity, but there may be some variation between individuals.
- Two-joint muscles play a role in movement at two joints. (Some muscles in the hand and foot cross more than two joints.) The most significant movements affected by two-joint muscles *and* spasticity **are indicated in orange** on the left side of the table.
- Typical ROMs for each joint are shown. The closer a joint's ROM is to typical, the better. A muscle contracture is a limitation of a joint's ROM.[93] The terms "muscle contracture" and "tight muscle" are used interchangeably in the CP field and in this book.

To stretch a muscle, we do the opposite of that muscle's action. To stretch a flexor muscle, for example, we must extend the joint. To stretch an extensor muscle, we must flex the joint.

To fully stretch a muscle, we must move the joint through its full ROM. Because some muscles cross two joints rather than one, both joints are involved in the stretching of two-jointed muscles. To stretch the two-jointed hamstrings, for example, we have to extend the knee while flexing the hip. Long sitting (sitting with the legs extended) is a good method of stretching the hamstrings because the knees are extended while the hips are flexed.

I compiled a version of this table many years ago, and it greatly helped my understanding of the condition. It came in handy when medical professionals referred to various movements or muscles or to a joint being tight (having a decreased ROM). I also found it helpful to be aware of the normal ROM for each joint. When surgery was planned, it helped me understand why procedures such as hip adductor and gastrocnemius lengthening were needed. For these reasons, it is worth taking some time to study this table. It will also be useful as a reference when reading later sections of this book.

Table 2.4.1 Lower limb movements, joint ROMs,[94,95] and key muscles

MOVEMENT (Green background indicates movements affected by spasticity)		KEY MUSCLES RESPONSIBLE FOR THE MOVEMENT (Two-jointed muscles are indicated in orange)
Hip flexion Movement of the thigh up toward the pelvis **ROM 0 to 125 degrees**		**Hip flexors** • Iliopsoas • Rectus femoris
Hip adduction Movement of the thigh toward the midline **ROM 0 to 20 degrees**		**Hip adductors** • Adductor longus • Adductor magnus • Adductor brevis • Gracilis
Hip internal rotation Rotary movement of the thigh toward the midline; also known as inward or medial rotation **ROM 0 to 45 degrees**	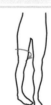	*Individual muscles not listed*
Knee flexion Increasing the angle between the thigh and lower leg **ROM 0 to 140 degrees** Note: Reference point is the straight leg. The angle increases the nearer the lower leg moves to the thigh.	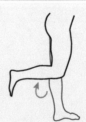	**Knee flexors** • Hamstrings • Gastrocnemius
Ankle plantar flexion Movement of the foot away from the lower leg **ROM 0 to 45 degrees** Note: Reference point is the 90-degree angle between the lower leg and the foot.	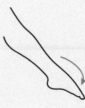	**Ankle plantar flexors** • Gastrocnemius • Soleus

OPPOSITE MOVEMENT		KEY MUSCLES RESPONSIBLE FOR THE OPPOSITE MOVEMENT
Hip extension Movement of the thigh away from the pelvis **ROM 0 to 10 degrees**	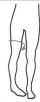	**Hip extensors** • Gluteus maximus • Hamstrings
Hip abduction Movement of the thigh away from the midline **ROM 0 to 45 degrees**		**Hip abductors** • Gluteus medius
Hip external rotation Rotary movement of the thigh away from the midline; also known as outward or lateral rotation **ROM 0 to 45 degrees**	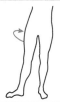	*Individual muscles not listed*
Knee extension Decreasing the angle between the thigh and lower leg **ROM 140 to 0 degrees** Note: Reference point is the flexed leg. The angle decreases the further the lower leg moves away from the thigh.		**Knee extensors** The quadriceps (quads) consist of four muscles: • Rectus femoris • Vastus intermedius • Vastus lateralis • Vastus medialis
Ankle dorsiflexion Movement of the foot toward the lower leg **ROM 0 to 20 degrees** Note: Reference point is the 90-degree angle between the lower leg and the foot.		**Ankle dorsiflexors** • Tibialis anterior • Toe extensors

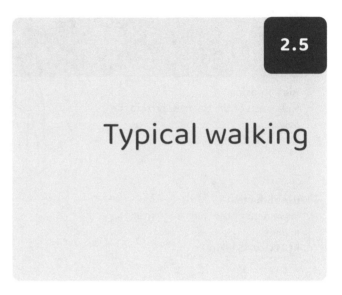

Typical walking

> A journey of a thousand miles begins with a single step.
>
> **Lao Tzu**

In general, we take walking for granted. It is only when we encounter a problem that we stop to think about what walking entails. The term "gait" refers to a person's manner of walking. "Typical" gait refers to the typically developing person's manner of walking, which has been studied extensively. Because having problems with walking is one of the hallmarks of spastic diplegia, this section briefly looks at the features of typical walking.

Walking is a phenomenal achievement. It involves generating forces, managing gravity, speed, balance, and more. In evolutionary terms, walking on two limbs was advantageous because it freed our upper limbs for other tasks. It is no surprise that crawling comes before walking in human gross motor development: a crawling child has four limbs on the floor and is therefore more stable. Walking, which involves balancing on two limbs, is a more advanced and more demanding form of movement.

The requirements of walking

Walking has four requirements:[96]

- **A control system:** The nervous system provides the control system for walking.
- **An energy source:** The energy required is supplied by oxygen[*] and the breakdown of food.
- **Levers providing movement:** The levers are the bones.
- **Forces to move the levers:** Muscle contraction provides the forces for walking. As we saw in the previous section, movement is generated by muscle forces acting on the levers (the bones).

The gait cycle

One complete gait (or walking) cycle refers to the time between two successive occurrences of the same event in walking—for example, the time between when one foot strikes the ground and when that same foot strikes the ground again. Figure 2.5.1 shows what is happening with each limb during a complete gait cycle. The gait cycle is divided into two major phases:

- **Stance phase:** The period of time the foot of interest (green in Figure 2.5.1) is on the ground
- **Swing phase:** The period of time the foot of interest is in the air

Stance phase occupies approximately 60 percent of the gait cycle, and swing phase occupies approximately 40 percent.[96] There are two periods in the gait cycle when both limbs are on the ground; this is termed "double stance" (or "double support"). Single stance (or single support) is when just one limb is on the ground. Walking involves alternately balancing on each single limb as we move forward.

---

[*] Energy can be produced without oxygen in some cases; for example, for short bursts of quick walking. This is termed "anaerobic metabolism."

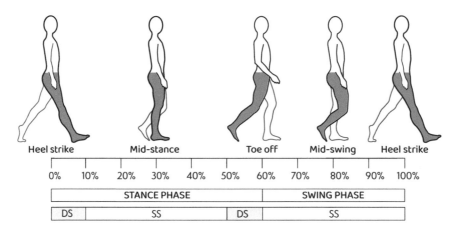

Figure 2.5.1 A complete gait cycle. "DS" is double stance; "SS" is single stance.

Attributes of typical walking

The following are attributes of typical walking that are frequently lost in individuals with spastic diplegia:[96]

- **Stability in the stance phase:** A reflection of controlled movement and good balance
- **Foot clearance in the swing phase:** Movement of the foot forward without dragging the toe
- **Pre-positioning of the foot for initial contact (heel strike):** Preparation of the foot to strike the ground with the heel (see Figure 2.5.1)
- **Adequate step length:** A sufficiently long step taken
- **Energy conservation:** Energy-efficient walking

Problems with the first four of these attributes contribute to problems with the fifth, the energy cost of walking.

When a typically developing child begins to walk, they do so without these attributes. The knees are relatively stiff and they walk with a wide base of support (i.e., the legs are far apart). But as the child develops balance and their motor system matures, their gait evolves toward the adult pattern, generally by about three and a half years of age.[97] It appears that walking is innate rather than learned, and it depends on the progressive maturing of the central nervous system.

Primary problems

Divide each difficulty into as many parts as is
feasible and necessary to resolve it.

René Descartes

The motor system or neuromusculoskeletal system involves the nervous system, muscles, bones, joints, and their related structures. Based
on clinical expertise, Gage proposed a useful framework for classifying the neuromusculoskeletal problems that occur in children with
spastic CP.[74,98] Problems are categorized into primary, secondary, and
tertiary problems:

- Primary problems are caused by the brain injury and are therefore
  present from when the brain injury occurred. Many are neurological problems but may also include alterations in the structure of the
  muscles themselves.
- Secondary problems develop over time in the growing child. They
  are problems of atypical muscle growth and bone development and
  are referred to as "growth problems."
- Tertiary problems are the "coping responses" that arise to compensate for or counteract the primary and secondary problems.

Classifying the problems of spastic diplegia in this way is helpful because:

- For families, it may aid in their understanding of the many problems encountered. The classification helps explain how and when the problems likely develop and change over time.
- For medical professionals, it is important to separate out the different problems to decide what can, cannot, and should not be treated, providing a road map for treatment.

A very useful tool for classifying the problems, which can sometimes be difficult to separate, is gait analysis.* Gait analysis is addressed in Chapter 3. This section covers primary problems, and the next two cover secondary and tertiary problems.

The primary neuromusculoskeletal problems are problems present from when the brain injury occurred. In general, the primary problems are difficult to change or improve. However, with diligent management, the impact of these primary problems can be minimized, and function can be maximized.

Understanding the primary (this section), secondary (next section, 2.7), and tertiary (section 2.8) problems and how they combine to affect gait (section 2.9) is key to understanding spastic diplegia. These sections are long, but they are worth reading in order to gain a full understanding of the condition. Your physical therapist or physician may be able to answer any questions you may have. It may also help to use Table 2.4.1 as a reference.

Understanding this classification really helped me understand what was going on in spastic diplegia. I found the problems difficult to understand in the first place, but I also had trouble grasping how the condition would change over time. This classification was first published in 1991 and it has stood the test of time.

---

* A measurement tool used to evaluate gait. Within gait analysis, multiple variables are evaluated using different measurement tools (see section 3.8).

The primary problems include the following, which are examined each in turn, adapted from Gage:[74,98,99]

- **Lack of selective motor control**
- **Poor balance**
- **Abnormal tone**
- **Muscle weakness**
- **Sensory problems**

Even though primary problems are discussed separately, the problems exist together and they trend in similar directions (the level of effect of one is mirrored in others plus, they can exacerbate one another). Primary problems should be evaluated and considered separately while recognizing that they may trend together. In other words, if impairment is greater in one area (e.g., selective motor control), it tends to be greater in other areas (e.g., weakness). In general, the severity of primary problems is a significant predictor of GMFCS level.

Lack of selective motor control

In simple terms, selective motor control refers to the ability to isolate a muscle or combination of muscles to produce a particular movement. This includes being able to contract a muscle without the opposite muscle contracting (which is termed "co-contraction"). For example, some cannot wink one of their eyes, no matter how hard they try because they do not have good selective motor control over the muscles responsible for winking. Another example is ankle dorsiflexion/plantar flexion (moving the foot up and down) without moving knees or hips. A child with spastic diplegia has problems with selective motor control and therefore has difficulty performing some movements.

Selective motor control can be checked by asking the child to perform certain movements, such as moving the foot up and down. Each limb and joint is tested separately. This evaluates whether the child:

- Can do the full movement in both directions
- Can do the movement without involving other body movements
- Can do the movement without doing a mirror movement, or other movement, in the same or the other limb

The severity and number of muscles affected by lack of selective motor control in spastic diplegia depends on the extent of the brain injury.

People with spastic diplegia typically demonstrate fairly good selective motor control at the hip, less control at the knee, and the least control at the ankle and foot.[99] The brain injury associated with spastic diplegia occurs in the tracts near the ventricles of the brain. Figure 2.2.1 shows that the tracts to the ankle are closer to the site of the injury than those to the knee, which in turn are closer than those to the hip. Thus, the distal muscles (those further from the trunk) are more involved than the proximal muscles (those nearer the trunk). In addition, from the standpoint of selective motor control, muscles that cross more than one joint are more severely involved than muscles that cross only one joint.[99]

Tommy has difficulty dorsiflexing his right foot (bringing his right foot up). When he tries to dorsiflex his right foot, a mirror movement automatically occurs in his left foot.

Poor balance

Balance is generally understood as the ability to not fall. More specifically, it's about controlling our body within our base of support.[100] Good balance is needed to be able to function in our environment.

About half of our body mass is in our trunk,[101] so good balance largely relies on controlling our trunk position within the support base whether we are lying, sitting, standing, or walking. When we are lying down, our whole body is in contact with the surface, so balance is easy. When we are standing or walking, only our feet are in contact with the surface (ground), so balance is more challenging.

To control our body position, we also must sense where our body is and then move as appropriate. This means our motor and sensory systems are involved in balance. The motor system is the neuromusculoskeletal system already described, including the nervous system, muscles, bones, joints, and their related structures. Sensory systems involved include vision, vestibular input, proprioception, and tactile feedback:[102]

- Vision involves sensory receptors in our eyes.
- Vestibular input involves sensory receptors in our ears.
- Proprioception involves sensory receptors in our muscles and joints.
- Tactile feedback involves sensory receptors in our skin.

Our brain combines the information from all these sensory receptors to interpret our body position and motion relative to itself and our surroundings.[102] Individuals with CP, including those with spastic diplegia, may have deficits in one or more of the sensory or motor systems, any of which can impact balance.[3,103]

A gentle push (forward, backward and/or side to side) of a child tests balance reactions. A child with typical balance will easily maintain their balance and, if necessary, take a compensatory step to regain it. A child with balance problems may fall over or take longer to regain their balance (more than one step). In spastic diplegia, the child often falls backward due to poor posterior balance. These balance problems can be seen when balance is challenged (even in children with mild spastic diplegia), such as when the person tries to avoid an object or quickly changes direction.

Conflicting views exist in the literature on whether poor balance reactions can be improved by training and/or therapy.[103]

Tommy also has some balance problems; he was prone to falling backward when he was younger. Balance is still a challenge in adulthood.

Abnormal tone

Muscle tone is the resting tension in a muscle. A range of "normal" muscle tone exists. Tone is considered "abnormal" when it falls outside the range of normal or typical. It can be too low (hypotonia) or too high (hypertonia). Abnormal muscle tone occurs in all types of CP. In children with spastic diplegia, tone is typically too high in the legs and arms due to spasticity, but it can be low in the trunk.

a) Spasticity

Spasticity is one type of high tone. There are several definitions of spasticity. One is that it is a condition in which there is an abnormal increase in muscle tone or stiffness of muscle that can interfere with movement and speech, and be associated with discomfort or pain.[22] Another definition highlights the velocity-dependent nature of spasticity.[104]

A muscle reacts to rapid stretching by contracting in opposition (i.e., the muscle tightens rather than continuing to stretch or lengthen). This protects the muscle from overstretching when quickly stretched. See Figure 2.6.1.

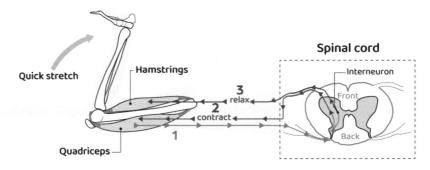

Figure 2.6.1 Example of a "normal" stretch reflex. **1.** Quadriceps are stretched quickly, and information is sent via sensory neurons to the spinal cord. **2.** Motor neurons cause the quadriceps to contract to resist the quick stretch. **3.** Motor neurons cause the hamstrings to relax to allow the quadriceps to contract.

- A **"normal" stretch reflex** is a rapid, involuntary muscle contraction (in the quadriceps in Figure 2.6.1) in response to a sudden stretch of the muscle.*
- A **"hyperactive" stretch reflex** is an exaggerated reflex response that leads to excessive muscle contraction and increased muscle tone. Spasticity is a hyperactive stretch reflex (the excessive muscle contraction can be felt as resistance by a person doing a quick passive stretch of the muscle).†

---

* Doctors routinely perform a knee-jerk reflex test using a small rubber hammer to check for healthy reflex responses.

† Passive stretching is when another person stretches an individual's muscle.

The speed of the rapid stretch is important because the spastic reaction happens only with a *quick* stretch. If the stretch is slow, it does not elicit a spastic reaction. (The effect of speed can be noted by comparing a muscle's response to slow versus quick passive stretching.) The muscle stretching that occurs, during walking for example, is quick (an entire gait cycle occurs in about one second); thus, the spastic response can happen in people with spastic diplegia while walking.

Spasticity results from a loss of inhibition—the dampening input from specific nerve cells in the brain to nerve cells in the spinal cord, and hence to certain muscles.

Clonus is the most extreme form of spasticity, defined as a series of involuntary, rhythmic muscular contractions and relaxations. It can be seen in the gastrocnemius (one of the calf muscles); for example, when an examiner quickly dorsiflexes the foot (moves the foot up), the foot may then plantar flex (move down) and continue to move up and down uncontrollably for a number of beats (contraction and relaxation cycles). A video depicting clonus is included in **Useful web resources.**

b) Dystonia

As noted in section 2.1, individuals with spastic diplegia sometimes have secondary or co-occurring motor types in addition to spasticity. The Australian CP register found that 12 percent of individuals with spastic diplegia (all GMFCS levels) have co-occurring dyskinesia.[*][42] It is believed that the true prevalence of co-occurring motor types is higher.[4] A more recent study found that 50 percent of children and young people with CP had spasticity *and* dystonia.[48] The presence of dystonia with spasticity has been underrecognized, which is important to note because the management of spasticity and dystonia is different.

Dystonia is a disorder characterized by involuntary (unintended) muscle contractions that cause slow repetitive movements or abnormal postures that can sometimes be painful.[39] Some define dystonia as muscles that "contract that you do not want to contract when you try to move." In contrast to spasticity, dystonia does not occur as a result of rapid stretch. Examples of dystonia include the leg muscles tightening

---

* For those who acquired CP in the prenatal or perinatal period only.

or uncontrolled, posturing movements of the fingers or toes when surprised, talking, or playing a video game (where there is excitement or tension).

Abnormal muscle tone can be measured using different measurement tools. See Table 2.6.1.

Table 2.6.1 Measurement tools for abnormal muscle tone

MEASUREMENT TOOL	TYPE OF ABNORMAL MUSCLE TONE
Modified Ashworth Scale (MAS) [105,106]	Spasticity
Modified Tardieu Scale (MTS) [106,107]	Spasticity
Barry-Albright Dystonia Scale (BADS)[108]	Dystonia
Hypertonia Assessment Tool (HAT)[109,110]	Dystonia and spasticity (and rigidity*)

* Rigidity is another type of high tone in which the muscles have the same amount of stiffness irrespective of the degree of movement. It is uncommon and practically does not exist in CP.

Tommy has spasticity but also some dystonia.

Muscle weakness

In general terms, muscle weakness is the inability to generate muscle force. (Refer to Table 2.4.1, which shows the main lower limb muscles arranged in pairs around each joint.) A study found that the strength of the major muscle groups of both legs in children with spastic diplegia was less than that of those of age-matched typically developing peers.[111] The causes of the muscle weakness resulting from the brain injury are varied and include:

• Smaller muscles[112]
• Atypical muscle composition (i.e., more fat and collagen)[113]
• Poor selective motor control or co-contraction of muscles on the opposite side of the joint[3]
• Incomplete voluntary activation of the muscle[114]

- Decreased muscle lever arms, often due to bony malalignments or related problems[115,116,117]

Muscle strength can be measured by manual muscle testing, by a hand-held machine called a dynamometer, or with more sophisticated tests as might be done in a sports clinic. Measuring muscle strength for people with CP is challenging because of the lack of selective motor control and contractures.

> Muscle weakness in the major muscle groups of both legs is a problem for Tommy.

Sensory problems

A full discussion of sensory problems is included in section 2.10.

Secondary problems

Just as the twig is bent the tree's inclined.
Alexander Pope

The secondary problems in spastic diplegia develop slowly over time and in direct proportion to the rate of bone growth. They also depend on the amount and type of usage of the muscles. We saw earlier that the periods of most rapid growth are from birth to age three and during puberty. These are, therefore, periods of great challenge and change in the child with spastic diplegia.

Secondary problems arise as a result of the atypical forces imposed on the growing skeleton by the effects of the primary brain injury and movement. In other words, the primary problems drive the secondary problems. The good news is that the secondary problems have more treatment options.

This section covers:

- **Atypical muscle growth**
- **Atypical bone development**

Atypical muscle growth

What follows is a simplified explanation of atypical muscle growth in spastic diplegia. This is a very complex subject, and more is still being learned about the differences between muscles in typically developing individuals and in people with spastic CP. Also, as noted in the last section, the primary problems may also include alterations in the structure of the muscles themselves. A muscle grows in length in response to stretch. It has been shown that for normal muscle lengthening to occur, two to four hours of stretching per day is required.[98] Bones grow during sleep,[118] and in a typically developing child, this required amount of stretching occurs when the child gets up in the morning and starts to move about, to run, and to play. This typical movement moves the joints and results in normal stretching of the muscles, which provides the stimulus for laying down new muscle cells and is how a muscle grows in length. Thus, bone growth leads to stretching of the muscle, which leads to the muscle growing in length.

Because the primary problems predominantly affect the neuromusculoskeletal systems in children with spastic diplegia, they usually have decreased physical activity levels compared to typically developing children.[119] The reduced amount of physical activity can then affect their capacity to actively stretch their muscles. Even with movement, the child with spastic diplegia may not fully stretch out their muscles through the typical ROM of the joints. Thus, the reduced stretching range for many muscles may become the norm.

As a result, the muscles fail to grow adequately in length and width* and contractures develop,† which result in joints having reduced ROM. Indeed, in the past, CP was called "short muscle disease," although it's worth noting that despite this title, the problem arises from muscles failing to grow in length and width rather than from becoming shortened. With lack of movement, the muscles also become stiff.

For young children with spastic diplegia, their muscles may still achieve full ROM when they are relaxed; for example, during sleep. Over time,

---

* Muscles also grow in width. Growth in width has been shown to be decreased as well.[120]

† More precisely, the contracture occurs in the muscle-tendon unit (MTU) and/or capsule of the joint, not just the muscle.

however, they may develop contracture, meaning that the full joint ROM cannot be achieved at any time. One study found decreasing ROM in the lower limb muscles in children with CP (43 percent bilateral) from age 2 to 14 years.[121]

Contractures particularly affect the two-joint* muscles.[3] They interfere with positioning and movement. For example, the young child may not be able to long sit comfortably because of hamstring contractures. Contractures may also interfere with the typical movements that lead to achieving gross motor milestones. Hamstring contractures may result in walking with flexed knees. Decreased mobility at any age may lead to activity limitation and reduced participation. Nordmark and colleagues described the nature of the problem: a decrease in ROM with age may result in decreased mobility, which in turn results in a further decrease in ROM—a vicious circle.[121]

In addition to the factors outlined above that may cause contractures to develop over time, there may be differences at a tissue level between the muscles of individuals with CP and those of the typical population. These differences include:[3,120,122,123,124]

- **Smaller muscles** in both diameter and length, which may partially explain muscle weakness
- **Lengthened and fewer sarcomeres** (the functional unit of contraction of a muscle), though the muscle itself is shortened, this could also contribute to muscle weakness
- **Muscles being stiffer,** which is believed to be caused by atypical extracellular matrix (the network surrounding the muscle cells, consisting of collagen, proteins, and more)
- **Decrease in the number of satellite cells,** which are responsible for the majority of muscle growth
- **Increased fat and collagen,** which could contribute to muscle weakness even if the muscle is the same size

In summary, muscle quality and size may be different. Muscles may become smaller (less muscle bulk) and stiffer (less elastic) compared with those of typically developing children. Smaller muscle size has been reported in children with spastic CP compared to typically developing

---

* Including multi-joint muscles.

children and in children as young as 15 months.[125,126] It is to be expected that the muscles of a 14-year-old with spastic CP would be very different from those of a 1-year-old with spastic CP. There is still more to learn about altered muscle composition in spastic CP.

To compensate for atypical muscle growth in a child with CP, parents have to ensure that their child gets adequate opportunity to stretch and move their spastic muscles. Traditionally, this included the parent doing daily slow stretches of the child's spastic muscles through their full ROM. (This is called passive stretching; the slow stretching does not elicit the spastic response.) However, passive stretching is no longer recommended in isolation. The current evidence places a greater emphasis on other methods of stretching, including positioning, orthoses, casting,* and especially active movement. Because of its importance, a detailed section on stretching is included in the next chapter. The aim is to keep full ROM for as long as possible to prevent contractures from developing to the greatest possible extent. Working on ROM is not something that can begin when the child is older. It has to start right at the time of diagnosis. However, despite best efforts, it is often inevitable that some contractures may develop.

The rate of development of contractures often mirrors the rate of growth of the child; that is, contractures tend to develop during periods of rapid growth (which is why keeping a growth chart is useful). While great attention needs to be paid to stretching and activity during periods of active growth, stretching is needed throughout childhood and adolescence. Even in the "quieter" growth years, the child will still gain height.

Note that the situation can be even more complicated. It is possible for some muscles to become too long in response to abnormal postures and movement. One example is crouch gait (persistent flexed-knee gait). The one-joint muscles responsible for upright posture and alignment (gluteus maximus, vasti, and soleus) are stretched repetitively and for prolonged periods of time during growth. As a result, they gradually

---

* Casting consists of stretching a muscle by applying a plaster of paris or a fiberglass cast; for example, a below-knee cast to stretch the tight gastrocnemius and/or soleus muscles (calf muscles) to hold the muscle in a position of maximum stretch. After a few days to one week, the cast can be removed. A series of casts is typically needed to gain the desired effect.

become too stretched, too long, and less effective in maintaining upright posture. This sequence can result in progressively worsening crouch gait.

When Tommy was a small child, passive stretching was given more prominence than it is today (though still in combination with positioning, orthoses, casting, and active movement). My husband and I did the daily passive stretching, and organizing a typical day often included deciding which of us would "do Tommy's stretches." Over the years, Tommy developed contractures in a number of muscles.

Atypical bone development

This section addresses:

a) Lever-arm dysfunction
b) Scoliosis
c) Bone health

a) Lever-arm dysfunction

Atypical bone development is interlinked with atypical muscle growth in spastic diplegia. The long bones of the body (the bones of the upper and lower limbs) grow in a particular area called the "growth plates" (see Figure 2.7.1), but it is the forces acting on the bones that play a part in their ultimate shape—termed "bone modeling."[99]

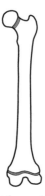

Figure 2.7.1 Growth plates (orange) in a long bone.

Growing bone is "plastic," or "malleable," which is what allows the forces to model the bone. The expressions "If you put a twist on a growing bone, it will take the twist" and "Just as the twig is bent the tree's inclined" illustrate this concept. If the muscle forces and bone forces are typical and occur at the correct time in development, then the final shape of the bone will be typical as well (e.g., the femoral head and the hip socket helping to shape each other). If forces are atypical or mistimed in relation to a child's development, the bones may be misshaped.

The movements that help the child achieve the six main gross motor milestones* described in Chapter 1 and the time in development at which they occur are part of the typical forces acting on the bones. It is important to understand that the bones of younger children are more malleable than the bones of older children. One of the hallmarks of spastic diplegia is that the child can be late in achieving gross motor milestones when the bones are less malleable with less ability to remodel or reshape. This is in addition to the influences of altered muscle forces and tone. We can compare this to providing opportunities for our children: we have to provide them at the right time. Peekaboo will delight your six-month-old infant, but your six-year-old child will likely roll their eyes if you try to play Peekaboo with them. In the presence of spastic diplegia, typical bone modeling (shaping) may not occur as the bone grows.

In addition to bone modeling, a certain amount of bone *remodeling* (reshaping) occurs in development.

The effectiveness of a muscle action to produce movement depends not only on the muscle but also on the shape and length of the bones and the position of the joints. If the position or shape of the bone and joint is not typical, the bone is less effective as a lever. For example, if the femur (thigh bone) is misshapen, the hip abductors cannot work as effectively because the pulling force of the muscle will be in an incorrect direction. Gage coined the term "lever-arm dysfunction" to describe the influence of bone problems on movement.[74] These problems include lever arms (bones) that are short, flexible, twisted, and/or in the wrong position.

---

* The milestones are significant, but so are the movements leading up to the milestones. For example, when a child is able to stand holding on to furniture, they may also be able to hold on with one hand and turn their body to bend down and pick up an object. All these movements, not just the main movements, contribute to the normal forces that act on the bones.

The following are common problems in spastic diplegia; each is explained below:

i) Hip displacement (subluxation and dislocation)
ii) Excessive femoral anteversion
iii) Tibial torsion
iv) Pes valgus

i) Hip displacement (subluxation and dislocation)

The hip joint is a ball-and-socket joint that is formed by the head (ball) of the femur and the acetabulum (socket) of the pelvis. Under the influence of bone growth and spastic muscles, a child's hip may become displaced: the ball moves partially out of the socket. This can be progressive and can lead to complete displacement. There are two stages of hip displacement:

- **Subluxated hip (hip subluxation)** is when the ball is partially out of the socket but is still in contact with it—the ball is still partially covered by the socket.
- **Dislocated hip (hip dislocation)** is when the ball has moved completely out of the socket.

The development of hip displacement is a slow process. Even though it starts out silently (it is painless), it can lead to pain and reduced function in the longer term. See Figure 2.7.2.

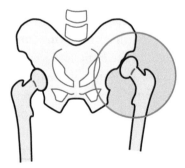

Figure 2.7.2 A dislocated hip. The right hip is normal. The left hip is dislocated: the head of the femur (ball) has moved completely out of the acetabulum (socket) of the pelvis.

Research has shown that the risk of hip displacement increases with GMFCS level.[127,128] The risk for children with CP has been found to be:

- The same as typically developing children for GMFCS level I
- 15 percent for GMFCS level II
- 41 percent for GMFCS level III

The measure used in X-rays for hip surveillance (monitoring) is called the "migration percentage" (MP), also known as the Reimer's migration index (RMI). Both terms refer to the percentage of the ball that has moved out of the socket, which can range from 0 to 100. "Normal" is less than 10 percent,[3] and hip displacement (subluxation) is anything greater than that. Mild abnormalities may not be problematic, but once the MP is greater than 30 percent, the likelihood of further displacement is almost certain (if there is growth remaining). Hip dislocation is defined as MP over 90 and up to 100 percent.[129]

See section 3.3 for more information on hip surveillance.

You may also come across the term "dysplasia," which means abnormal growth. Though closely related to hip displacement, it is not the same thing. Acetabular dysplasia is when the hip socket doesn't develop correctly and becomes shallow. It both results from and contributes to hip displacement.

ii) Excessive femoral anteversion
The important parts of the femur for the purposes of this discussion are the head (ball), neck, and shaft. The neck connects the head with the shaft. See Figure 2.7.3.

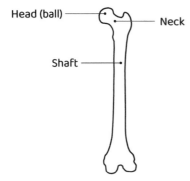

Figure 2.7.3 A femur.

The term "femoral anteversion" comes from "femoral" referring to the femur (thigh bone) and "version" referring to the angle of the neck of the femur relative to the shaft. "Ante" means "forward." "Femoral anteversion," therefore, is a condition where the neck of the femur is rotated relatively forward.

Figure 2.7.4 is a view of a hip and leg from the top down. The range of "normal" values for femoral anteversion varies depending on the reference used, but typically it's around 0 to 30 degrees in adults.[130,131] The mean value for adult females is 15 degrees and for men it's 10 degrees.

At birth, a typically developing infant has approximately 40 degrees of femoral anteversion.[132] With typical movement, the anteversion they have at birth rapidly decreases in the first three to four years and further reduces until puberty to typical adult values.

In children with spastic diplegia, femoral anteversion may not be corrected with growth. In fact, the femoral anteversion present at birth not only fails to reduce with growth but may increase. This is termed "excessive femoral anteversion."

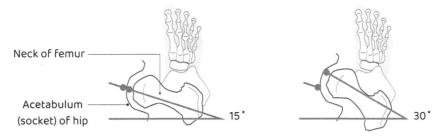

Figure 2.7.4 Femoral anteversion, top-down view: normal (left), with the neck of the femur correctly aligned with the acetabulum (socket) of the hip, and excessive (right), with the neck of the femur not correctly aligned.

The mean femoral anteversion for children with CP increases with GMFCS level and is:[128]

- 30 degrees for GMFCS level I
- 36 degrees for GMFCS level II
- 40 degrees for GMFCS level III

Excessive femoral anteversion often leads to walking with inward knee rotation and the foot turned in (intoeing). This helps the hip abductors be in a better position to act more effectively because it increases the muscle's lever arm. However, this turning in of the knee and foot leads to functional difficulties such as tripping and falling.

"Femoral torsion" means a twisted femur. While technically it is not the same as "femoral anteversion," the effect on function and treatment is similar, which is why the two terms are often used interchangeably.

iii) Tibial torsion

The tibia is the main bone in the lower leg, often called the shinbone. Tibial torsion is a twist in the tibia. At birth, the typically developing child has about five degrees of internal tibial torsion (i.e., an inward twist of the tibia).[133] As with the femur, with the right forces acting at the right time and in the right sequence, the internal tibial torsion present in the infant turns into 10 to 15 degrees of external tibial torsion in the adult.[134] However, in the child with spastic diplegia, the internal tibial torsion may not correct (persistent internal tibial torsion causing intoeing) or may overcorrect over time and become "excessive external" tibial torsion, with the foot turning out too much. See Figure 2.7.5.

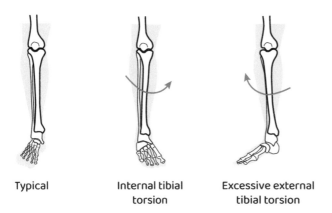

Typical | Internal tibial torsion | Excessive external tibial torsion

Figure 2.7.5 Tibial torsion of the right leg. Left: typical—foot exhibiting 10 to 15 degrees of external tibial torsion. Middle: internal tibial torsion—foot slightly turned in. Right: excessive external tibial torsion—foot excessively turned out.

The internal tibial torsion present at birth sometimes persists in children with spastic diplegia, but, as noted above, it often develops into an excessive external twist. Persistent internal tibial torsion may be seen in the younger child with spastic diplegia, while excessive external tibial torsion may be seen in the older child with spastic diplegia.

It is worth noting that in a child with femoral torsion *and* external tibial torsion, the femur (upper leg) is turned inward, but the tibia (lower leg) is turned outward.

iv) Pes valgus
The term "pes valgus" originates from "pes," meaning foot, and "valgus," meaning turning away from midline. Pes valgus is a series of complex hindfoot, midfoot, and forefoot malalignments. (The hindfoot is the heel. The midfoot is the middle of the foot around the arch. The forefoot comprises the toes and the long bones leading up to the toes). Table 2.7.1 explains the components of pes valgus.

The three segments of the foot develop malalignments over time in response to the atypical forces exerted on the bones, and they are commonly seen together. These malalignments reduce the effectiveness of the bones as lever arms and thus interfere with movement. Think of a person whose foot is turned outward as they attempt to walk forward. The foot needs to be stiff and extended in the last part of the stance phase of the gait cycle to propel the body forward. If the foot is too flexible, it becomes ineffective at doing its job. This is an example of a lever arm that is too flexible.

Table 2.7.1 Pes valgus

COMPONENT	ILLUSTRATION
Valgus hindfoot: The heel is turned outward from the midline of the body to an abnormal degree.	The left foot has a valgus hindfoot; the right foot is normal.
Pronation of the midfoot: This is a rotation of the bones on the inside of the arch at the midfoot so that in walking, the arch rolls inward to the floor.	The left foot has a pronated midfoot; the right foot is normal.
Abduction of the forefoot: The front of the foot is turned outward from the midline of the body to an abnormal degree.	The forefoot on the left is abducted; the forefoot on the right is typical.

You may also come across the term "equinovalgus." Equinovalgus includes the features of pes valgus, but a tightness in the calf muscle may cause a pull on the heel to raise it off the ground. The midfoot and forefoot remain on the ground when standing or walking. However, at its most extreme, this condition causes the individual to walk on their forefoot.

b) Scoliosis

Scoliosis is a three-dimensional rotation and curvature of the spine. When viewed from the back, the spine of a person with scoliosis is a C- or S-shaped curve instead of a straight line. See Figure 2.7.6.

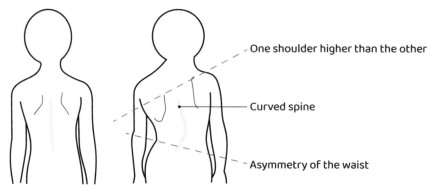

One shoulder higher than the other

Curved spine

Asymmetry of the waist

Figure 2.7.6 A typical spine (left) and a spine with scoliosis (right, showing a C-shaped curve). Note that one shoulder is higher than the other and there is asymmetry at the waist.

The angle of the scoliosis curve, the Cobb angle (also referred to as the curve magnitude) is measured on an X-ray image. The Cobb angle is the angle between the two most tilted vertebrae* at the upper and lower ends of a spinal curve (see Figure 2.7.7). A diagnosis of scoliosis is made when the Cobb angle is 10 degrees or greater. The Cobb angle is also used to monitor scoliosis progression and to guide treatment recommendations.

---

* The spine consists of vertebrae (the plural of vertebra) and intervertebral discs. Vertebrae are bony structures with a hole in the middle for the spinal cord to pass through.

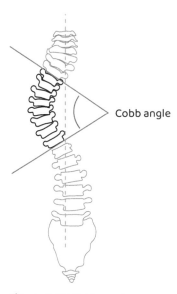
Cobb angle

Figure 2.7.7 Cobb angle measurement.

The prevalence and severity of scoliosis in individuals with CP increases with GMFCS level.[135,136] The prevalence of scoliosis was found to be:[136]

- 14 percent for GMFCS level I
- 15 percent for GMFCS level II
- 42 percent for GMFCS level III

However, for those with CP GMFCS levels I to III, most scoliosis curves are small, mostly nonprogressive, and with minimal or no symptoms.[136]

c) Bone health

Bone is a living tissue that is constantly being created, removed, and replaced. The term "osteoporosis" means "porous bones" (i.e., bones with low bone density*). Low bone density arises when either insufficient new bone is created or the rate of absorption of bone is greater than the rate of formation.

As people age, more bone is naturally lost than replaced. People with osteoporosis, however, have greater bone loss than is normal for their

---

* The terms "bone density" and "bone mineral density" are used interchangeably.

age. Figure 2.7.8 shows a normal bone and one with osteoporosis; the latter has much less bone material (i.e., less bone density).

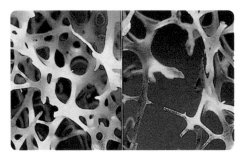

Figure 2.7.8 Cross-section of normal (left) and osteoporotic bone (right). Reproduced from Wikipedia user Gtirouflet, used under a Creative Commons license.

Bones can become so weak that a break (fracture) may occur with stress (such as a fall). A break may even occur spontaneously. Osteoporosis is a "silent" disease in that it is often diagnosed only when a bone fracture occurs. It is the most common cause of bone fractures among elderly people.

"Osteopenia" is the term used to define bone density that is not normal but not as low as in osteoporosis.[137] It can be regarded as the midpoint between healthy bone and osteoporosis. Having osteopenia places a person at risk of developing osteoporosis.

Bone health is determined by measuring bone mineral density (BMD) with a Z-score, which represents the number of standard deviations* an individual's bone density differs from the average for their age and sex. The cutoff for low bone density is a Z-score of -2.0. A study of BMD levels in children with CP (all subtypes) found evidence of low BMD for those at GMFCS levels II and III but not GMFCS level I.[138] The study also found that approximately two-thirds of the children (all CP subtypes and all GMFCS levels) had insufficient vitamin D, which is important for calcium metabolism in the body and for bone development.[138]

---

* The extent to which a point differs from the mean or average.

As a snapshot in time, Tommy's secondary problems at age nine included:

- Reduced ROM in many joints (both sides)
- Excessive femoral anteversion (right side)
- Excessive external tibial torsion (right side)
- Pronation of the midfoot (both sides)

Tertiary problems

Our greatest glory is not in never falling,
but in rising every time we fall.
Confucius

The tertiary problems in spastic diplegia are the coping responses or compensations that arise due to the individual's need to deal with or get around the primary and secondary problems.[99] Following are some examples of tertiary problems that may arise in spastic diplegia:

- **Pelvic obliquity:** One hip being higher than the other when viewed from the front. This may be the result of the individual being up on the toes of one side more than the other (asymmetric equinus). The asymmetry at the feet causes the hips to be at different levels.
- **Truncal sway (also referred to as trunk sway):** A side-to-side swaying of the trunk in walking, generally a compensation for hip abductor weakness.
- **Retracted pelvis:** Walking with the pelvis on one side rotated back (retracted) and rotated forward on the other side (protracted).

- **Vaulting:** Rising up on the toes during stance on one side in order to help clear the other leg during swing. The term "vault" means "jump" or "leap over." Vaulting is a common compensation and can be mistaken as a primary or secondary problem.

To correct the tertiary problems, the root cause (i.e., the primary and secondary problems), not the compensation, needs to be addressed. In the case of truncal sway, for example, addressing hip abductor weakness may reduce the sway.

While compensations are often the most visually apparent features of CP, they do not require treatment; these compensations—the tertiary problems—may be reduced or eliminated when the underlying cause is treated and they are no longer required.*[99]

> Tommy's tertiary problems at age nine included both pelvic obliquity and truncal sway.

---

* It is worth noting that these compensations are general gait compensations that may be found in other disabilities, not just CP.

Walking in individuals with spastic diplegia

I get up. I walk. I fall down. Meanwhile I keep dancing.
Daniel Hillel

The manner in which a person with spastic diplegia walks results from a combination of the neurological problems present from birth (the primary problems), the muscle and bone problems that develop with growth (the secondary problems), and any coping responses that develop as a result (the tertiary problems).

In a typically developing child, once mature walking has developed by around three and a half years of age,[97] their manner of walking changes little. The development of mature walking takes longer in children with CP and is dependent on GMFCS level. The gait of a person with spastic diplegia may also change over time as growth occurs and more atypical muscle and bone problems accumulate.

Rodda and colleagues classified the gait patterns seen in spastic diplegia, identifying four groups with increasing severity, from group I, true equinus, in which the child walks on their toes but with extended hips and knees, to group IV, in which the child walks in crouch gait (persistent flexed-knee gait).[*][139] This classification shows how progression or deterioration of gait may occur over time. It is important to remember, however, that not all children with spastic diplegia develop crouch gait. We address crouch gait in detail in this section.

A video explaining different gait patterns is included in **Useful web resources.**

We saw in section 2.5 that energy conservation is one of the five attributes of typical walking. Walking with spastic diplegia is less energy efficient than typical walking. Think of energy expenditure during walking like the fuel efficiency of a car. A more efficient car will consume less fuel while traveling a set distance. People can generate energy at a finite rate. A person with spastic diplegia, with their energy-inefficient gait, travels a shorter distance for a given amount of energy or gets tired more easily when they have to walk a set distance. This has important consequences for activity and participation.

For a child with spastic diplegia, walking is roughly as demanding as climbing stairs would be for a typically developing child. This is why fatigue is common in people with spastic diplegia. A study of 573 individuals with bilateral CP found that oxygen consumption during gait, a measure of energy expenditure, was 2.9 times that of speed-matched typically developing peers.[140] Can the child, adolescent, or young adult keep up with their peers in terms of speed or the distance they cover? Do they frequently feel fatigued and need to rest? All the factors that cause the increased energy expenditure of walking for all children with CP are not yet fully understood.

Gait problems generally increase with increasing GMFCS level. Studies have shown a higher prevalence[141] and greater severity[142] of gait problems

---

* The Rodda et al. classification is as follows:[139]
  - Group I: True equinus. The child is walking on their toes but with extended hips and knees. It is commonly seen in younger children when they first learn to walk.
  - Group II: Jump gait. Characterized by toe walking (equinus) and some degree of flexion at the knee and hip. It is the most common pattern in the preadolescent.
  - Group III: Apparent equinus. The child walks on their toes, though they still have full ROM in their ankle joints, hence the term "apparent." This is often a transitional stage, as the majority of children go on to develop crouch gait.
  - Group IV: Crouch gait (explained in this section). Some people might regard groups II and III as forms of crouch gait.

with increasing GMFCS level. However, the authors of one of these studies[142] also found there was a wide variation in gait problems within GMFCS levels; thus, GMFCS level is not a useful guide to gait problems. Two children at GMFCS level II, for example, could have very different gaits: one could be walking relatively erect but the other could be walking in crouch.

Three longitudinal studies of gait in children and adolescents showed deterioration in gait over time in untreated spastic diplegia[143,144,145] (the outcome of an untreated condition is known as the natural history of the condition). The time interval for deterioration was as low as 1.5 years. These studies underscore the importance of treating gait problems.

Three-dimensional (3D) computerized motion analysis is a very important tool for understanding the gait deviations that arise in spastic diplegia and for planning treatment, and is addressed in Chapter 3. Two children with spastic diplegia may walk similarly, but the mechanisms behind their walking may differ, and 3D computerized motion analysis helps understand each child's gait and the problems contributing to it.

Crouch gait

Because crouch gait is one of the most prevalent and functional gait problems seen in spastic diplegia, it is addressed in detail here. Crouch gait can be defined as persistent flexed-knee gait. It looks like a person placed their hand on the child and pushed them downward. The child flexes at both the hips and the knees. The child stands and walks with this posture. See Figure 2.9.1.

The exact degree of knee flexion that constitutes crouch gait varies in the literature but is typically greater than or equal to 20 degrees. This knee flexion is normally also accompanied by persistent hip flexion. The foot position can be variable; it can either be in plantar flexion (the child is on their toes) or dorsiflexion (the child has flat feet and flexed knees). Crouch gait may progress as the child grows. It should be thought of as a continuum from mild to severe.

Stout and colleagues classified crouch gait as follows:[146]

- **Mild crouch:** Typically seen in the younger child. This may be associated with internal hip rotation and the child being in equinus (up on their toes).
- **Moderate crouch:** Typically seen in adolescence in the person who has been walking in this posture for longer, and hamstring contracture may have developed.
- **Severe crouch:** Typically seen in older children.

This classification is similar to other classification systems.[139,147]

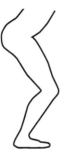

Figure 2.9.1 Crouch gait.

There are many problems associated with crouch gait, particularly when it becomes severe:

- It can worsen with time and lead to decreasing or loss of walking ability.
- Knee pain, caused by pressure on the kneecap (chondromalacia*), may decrease walking ability.
- Fracture of the patella (kneecap) may be present.
- Back pain may be a problem.
- It may affect the child's or adolescent's self-image and confidence.

Crouch gait may be caused by a number (and any combination) of factors, including:

- Hip flexion contractures or tightness (secondary problem)
- Knee flexion contractures or tightness (secondary problem)
- Weak antigravity muscles (primary and secondary problems)

---

* A condition in which the cartilage on the undersurface of the patella deteriorates and softens. It can be painful.

- Any treatment that excessively weakens the ankle plantar flexors (soleus/gastrocnemius)
- Lever-arm problems; that is, bone problems (secondary problem)
- Problems with balance and selective motor control (primary problem)

The antigravity muscles (those that resist or counteract gravity) that contribute to extension posture are the hip extensors, knee extensors, and ankle plantar flexors (see Table 2.4.1). In spastic diplegia, it is mainly the hip extensors and ankle plantar flexors that are weak. Keeping adequate strength in these muscle groups is important, especially for the ankle plantar flexors because they make a significant contribution to extension posture—although, for most people with spastic diplegia, the neurological deficits substantially limit what is actually possible. The plantar flexors (particularly the soleus) control the tibia (shin bone); they pull the tibia back to straighten (extend) the knee.

The mechanics of crouch gait are complicated. When standing, gravity acts on the body to exert a downward force, while an opposite upward force is produced by the ground. The latter is called the ground reaction force (GRF).[*] The position and shape of the body and body parts determine where the GRF acts on the joints and the muscles or positions that are required to counteract it:

- When standing with extended knees (i.e., with knees straight), the GRF acts in front of the knees and helps keep them extended (straight). This is useful because less muscle action is required to keep the knees extended.
- When standing with knees excessively flexed, the GRF moves behind the knees and causes a flexion force. This results in the antigravity muscles having to work much harder to resist the GRF, which is acting to collapse the knees. See Figure 2.9.2.

---

[*] Consider a box on the floor. The GRF from the floor is sufficient to oppose the pull of gravity on the box. Now, imagine a paper bag with handles, and put a heavy object in it. The reaction force of the bag is not sufficient (does not have enough resistance) against the heavy object, which bursts through the bottom of the bag and falls out. The pull of gravity on the object is stronger than the reaction force from the bag; thus, the bag cannot support the object.

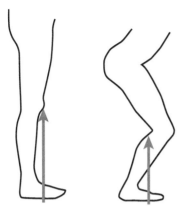

Figure 2.9.2 Position of ground reaction force (GRF) in relation to the knee. Left: The GRF acts in front of the knees and helps keep them extended (straight). Right: The GRF is behind the knees and causes a flexion force.

If the plantar flexors have been weakened, they cannot function effectively to straighten the knee (by pulling the tibia back) in standing or walking; thus, the knee extensors and hip extensors have to work harder to keep the body erect. Because of the flexed knees in crouch gait, this "free" extension force (when the ground reaction force falls in front of the knee) is lost. Gage coined the term "plantar flexor/knee extension couple," referring to the concept that the plantar flexors can extend the knee.[74]

Once crouch starts to develop, it can become self-perpetuating. Walking continuously in a flexed pattern means that:

• Certain muscles may be continuously in a shortened state, causing contractures.
• Other muscle-tendon units are continuously in a lengthened state, becoming overlengthened. This particularly affects the patellar tendon (the tendon that connects the kneecap, or patella, to the tibia).

In section 2.4, we saw that muscles generate optimal force when operating in the middle of the muscle's resting length (i.e., when the muscle is neither too short nor too long). Muscles that are overshortened (with contractures) or overlengthened are not as effective at generating force. It's like trying to get a child to operate a seesaw but placing them closer to the center of the apparatus. No matter how hard they try, they will not be able to generate sufficient force to make their side of the seesaw go down. The same occurs in spastic diplegia, except here the muscles may have multiple disadvantages (they may be excessively short, excessively long, spastic, and/or weak) and may be trying to exert that force on a bone that may itself not be typical (in shape and/or position).

As a child grows, the rate of increase in body mass* is far higher than the rate of increase in muscle strength. This is because body mass, which is related to volume, increases as a function of the cube law, but muscle strength, which is related to the cross-sectional area of the muscles, only increases as a function of the square.†

The unfavorable strength-to-mass ratio that develops as a child grows may exacerbate an already-developing crouch gait. Young children are relatively strong for their mass, but as they grow, their muscle strength may not keep pace. Thus, crouch often gets worse as the child gains mass. (This strength-to-mass ratio change applies to all children and adolescents, not just those with spastic diplegia. It just goes unnoticed in typically developing children because their muscles are sufficiently strong.) It is therefore very important for the child with spastic diplegia to have maximal muscle strength as they grow. Preserving plantar flexor strength and maintaining an effective plantar flexor/knee extension couple is important for preventing crouch gait.

Although crouch gait is common in spastic diplegia, it is complex and professionals are still learning about it and may not yet fully understand all the factors that contribute to it.

---

* There is a subtle difference between mass and weight. Mass is the actual amount of material in an object, measured in kilograms or pounds. Weight is the force exerted by gravity on that object. Weight is different on Earth than it is on the moon (where gravity is one-sixth of that on Earth), whereas mass is the same on both.

† Here is a very simple example to illustrate the point. A young child has a body mass of 2 units and muscle strength of 2 units. If body mass increases as a function of the cube but muscle strength increases as a function of the square, then after a number of years, the older child's body mass will be 8 units (2 x 2 x 2), whereas their muscle strength will be 4 units (2 x 2). The older child has much less muscle strength for their body mass than the younger child.

At age nine, Tommy walked with moderate crouch gait. His oxygen consumption while walking was 2.5 times normal, meaning his walking was two and a half times more energy demanding than it was for his peers.

Gait analysis helped identify his particular problems at that point in time and develop a tailored treatment plan. The logical classification of his problems and the ensuing treatment plan to address them gave us confidence that this was the correct path to follow.

Associated problems

Create the highest, grandest vision possible for your life,
because you become what you believe.

Oprah Winfrey

We have addressed the neuromusculoskeletal issues that arise in spastic diplegia and their effects on motor function. In section 2.1, we saw that a minority of children with spastic diplegia (all GMFCS levels) have problems in the areas of speech, intelligence (cognition), epilepsy, vision, and hearing of varying severity. However, more than 90 percent of children have none or only one severe associated problem.[80] The prevalence and severity of associated problems have been found to be greater in children at higher GMFCS levels compared with those at lower GMFCS levels.[80]

This section looks at associated problems that children and adolescents with spastic diplegia may have. These problems are important to consider because for some individuals with spastic diplegia, they may reduce their well-being far more than any of their motor problems.

- **Speech, language, communication, and feeding:** Approximately one in two children with spastic diplegia have some level of speech challenge.[80] Due to the motor, sensory, and cognitive problems caused by the brain injury, children may have difficulties with:

  o Oral motor movements[*] that affect speech production, including imprecise articulation[†] and slowed speech production
  o Respiratory strength or control affecting voice or speech loudness
  o Manipulation of food and swallowing

  These problems, if present, can range from mild to severe. Associated conditions such as hearing problems and seizures can further impact speech and swallowing skills.

- **Sensory problems:** "Sensory" refers to the senses that include vision, hearing, taste, smell, and touch. "Sensation" can be defined as the physical feeling or perception arising from something that happens to or that comes in contact with the body. "Decreased sensation" means a reduction in the ability to perceive sensory stimuli. "Tactile problems" are ones related to the sense of touch. Sensory input gives us much information about the outside world, which we then incorporate into learning and actions.

  Approximately one in three children with spastic diplegia has some level of **vision** challenge.[80] Strabismus, where the eyes do not look in the same direction at the same time, is more common among individuals with CP than in the typical population.[148] (Strabismus is often referred to as having crossed eyes or a squint.)

  Approximately 1 in 10 children with spastic diplegia has some level of **hearing** challenge.[80]

  Sensory problems can also include the inability to sense where a limb is in space (**proprioception**), and the inability to identify an object by feeling it (**stereognosis**).

---

* These relate to the muscles and structures involved in speech and other oral (mouth related) tasks; for example, chewing and swallowing.

† Production of clear and distinct sounds.

Sensory challenges can also include **cold extremities**. This can affect hands and feet, and for many it can be independent of ambient temperature. Fifty-six percent of ambulatory (able to walk) children with CP (all subtypes) reported cold extremities.[149] In some individuals, temperature changes can be associated with color changes of the hand and arm.

- **Epilepsy:** Just less than one in five children with spastic diplegia has epilepsy.[80] Epilepsy can be diagnosed if an individual experiences at least two unprovoked seizures (not stemming from any identifiable cause such as illness or fever) occurring more than 24 hours apart. A seizure is "uncontrolled, abnormal electrical activity of the brain that may cause changes in the level of consciousness, behavior, memory, or feelings."[150]

- **Pain:** Pain has been extensively reported in individuals with CP. Forty-eight percent of ambulatory children with CP (all subtypes) reported pain.[149] Common causes in children with CP include hip displacement, muscle spasms, procedures, headaches, neuropathic pain,[*] and visceral pain.[†151] Pain in childhood *or* adolescence has been strongly associated with low quality of life.[152,153]

- **Urinary and bowel continence:** A UK study found that children with bilateral CP GMFCS levels I to III achieved day and nighttime bowel and bladder continence more slowly and less completely than typically developing peers.[154] (See Table 2.10.1.) Attainment of continence decreased with increasing GMFCS level.

---

[*] A type of chronic pain caused by damage to the nervous system. It can be experienced as a burning or stabbing sensation unrelated to any external stimulus.

[†] A type of pain in the internal organs. It can be experienced as a dull, aching, or cramp-like pain and is difficult to precisely locate.

Table 2.10.1 Percentage of children with bilateral CP GMFCS levels I to III achieving day and nighttime bowel and bladder continence

GMFCS LEVEL	PERCENTAGE ACHIEVING BOWEL CONTINENCE		PERCENTAGE ACHIEVING BLADDER CONTINENCE	
	By day	By night	By day	By night
I	100% by day by age 5.5 years and by night by age 7 years			
II	95% by age 5 years	90% by age 5.5 years	96% by age 5 years	90% by age 5.5 years
III	74% by age 7 years	67% by age 9 years	65% by age 7 years	67% by age 9 years

Symptomatic neurogenic bladder (SNB) is a condition where there is dysfunction in the nerves controlling the bladder, leading to problems with urine storage and release. A US study found that 21 percent of individuals with spastic diplegia had SNB. Symptoms included incontinence, both day and nighttime, followed by urgency (sudden compelling need to urinate) and frequency (need to void at intervals less than two hours apart).[91]

- **Constipation:** Twenty-two percent of ambulatory children with CP (all subtypes) reported constipation.[149]

- **Sleep:** Sleep problems have been reported in 36 percent of ambulatory children with CP (all subtypes).[149] They include delayed insomnia, disrupted sleep, early awakening, or a combination. Suggested causes include difficulty to relax and calm down or presence of spasticity, anxiety, epilepsy, and pain.[149]

- **Cognition:** Approximately two in five children with spastic diplegia have some level of cognitive challenge.[80] Children may have difficulties related to processing, comprehension, learning, attention, expressive language, memory, organization, and problem-solving. To help identify and better understand specific cognitive or behavioral challenges, individuals with CP may be referred for neuropsychological evaluation.[*] This testing is valuable in identifying individual strengths and needs associated with coordinated brain functioning, assisting with securing additional resources and interventions as needed, and following progress over time or changes after interventions.

- **Sexual relationships:** Young adults with CP (51 percent bilateral, 93 percent GMFCS levels I to III, 18 to 22 years, average intelligence) had less experience in romantic and sexual relationships than their age-matched peers.[155] In addition, young adults with CP (51 percent bilateral, 89 percent GMFCS levels I to III, 20 to 24 years, average intelligence) experienced various problems or challenges with sexual relationships, including inability to achieve orgasm (20 percent), physical problems with sex[†] related to CP (80 percent), and emotional inhibition to initiate sexual contact (45 percent). Many have reported wanting information, including on the impact of CP on sexual function and fertility.[156]

- **Quality of life:** Quality of life (QOL) is defined as "the individual's perception of their position in life in the context of the culture and value system in which they live, and in relation to their goals, expectations, standards, and concerns."[157] A large European QOL study of 500 children with CP (47 percent bilateral spastic, 87 percent GMFCS levels I to III) age 8 to 12, who could self-report, found they have similar QOL to their peers.[152] A follow-up study of 431 adolescents with CP (all subtypes) age 13 to 17 found that they had significantly lower QOL than the general population in only 1 of the 10 domains measured—social support and peers[153]—and that adolescents with CP need help to maintain and develop peer relationships.[153]

Looking at the severity of impairments for children with CP:[152]

---

[*] Neuropsychology is a specialty that focuses on understanding brain functioning as it relates to cognition and behavior. Neuropsychological testing helps evaluate broad areas of cognitive function; for example, intelligence, language, visuospatial function, executive function, attention, memory, and processing speed. These areas frequently work in collaboration for efficient cognitive functioning.

[†] Includes spasticity, difficulty positioning, stiffness of joints and muscles, and fatigue.

○ Children with poorer walking ability had poorer *physical well-being.*

○ Those with intellectual impairment had lower *moods and emotions* and less *autonomy.*

○ Those with speech difficulty had poorer *relationships with their parents.*

Among adolescents with CP, severity of impairment was significantly associated with reduced QOL for moods and emotions, autonomy, and social support and peers.[153] Pain in childhood or adolescence was also strongly associated with low QOL.[152,153]

- **Mental and behavioral health**: Mental health has been defined as "a state of mental well-being that enables people to cope with the stresses of life, realize their abilities, learn well and work well, and contribute to their community."[158] While mental and behavioral health are closely related, they are different. Mental health has more to do with thoughts and emotions. Behavioral health has more to do with how people react in a situation—two people in the same situation may react in very different ways. Both mental and behavioral health strongly contribute to QOL.

The QOL study noted above observed no differences between children and adolescents with CP and peers in psychological well-being and moods and emotions (aspects of mental health). However, a number of studies have reported a higher level of mental health problems among children and adolescents with CP.[159,160,161]

  ○ A 2018 review of studies concluded that mental health symptoms are common in children and adolescents with CP. Those with an intellectual disability had a higher risk of mental health symptoms.[159]

  ○ A 2020 Danish study reported that the prevalence of mental health disorders was significantly higher in children and adolescents with CP (all subtypes) (22 percent) compared with peers (6 percent).[160]

  ○ Children and adolescents with CP (subtype not reported) experienced bullying and social exclusion at school and that this affects mental health.[161]

Noritz and colleagues suggested that the higher prevalence of mental and behavioral health problems in children and adolescents with CP may be due to the underlying brain injury, pain and physical difficulties, and limitations with participation.[162] It is important that problems with mental and behavioral health be addressed.

Key points Chapter 2

- With spastic diplegia, the lower limbs are much more affected than the upper limbs, which frequently show only fine motor impairment.
- Studies show that children with spastic diplegia have more problems with gross motor function—63 percent were functioning at GMFCS levels I and II while 76 percent were functioning at MACS levels I and II.
- Spasticity is the most common type of atypical tone present in individuals with spastic diplegia, although dystonia can be present as well.
- The classic brain injury of spastic diplegia is periventricular leukomalacia (PVL). The injury is usually bilateral (affecting both sides of the brain), but it can be uneven.
- A proportion of children with spastic diplegia (all GMFCS levels) have problems in the areas of speech, intelligence (cognition), vision, epilepsy, and hearing of varying severity. However, more than 90 percent of children have none or only one severe associated problem. These and other associated problems may reduce well-being far more than motor problems.
- A useful framework for classifying the musculoskeletal problems that occur in children with spastic CP categorizes them into primary, secondary, and tertiary problems. Primary problems are caused by the brain injury and are therefore present from when the brain injury occurred. Secondary problems develop over time in the growing child. They are problems of atypical muscle growth and bone development and are referred to as "growth problems." Tertiary problems are the "coping responses" that arise to compensate for or counteract the primary and secondary problems.
- A four-group classification system describes the gait patterns in individuals with spastic diplegia.
- Crouch gait, defined as persistent flexed-knee gait, is one of the most prevalent and functional gait problems seen in spastic diplegia and varies from mild to severe.

Chapter 3

Management and treatment of spastic diplegia to age 20

Introduction

Knowing is not enough; we must apply.
Willing is not enough; we must do.
Johann Wolfgang von Goethe

The difference between management and treatment is subtle. "Management" is the broader term, taking into account all aspects of an individual's life, whereas "treatment" refers to the use of a specific intervention; for example, physical therapy, orthoses, or orthopedic surgery. The terms "treatment" and "intervention" are largely interchangeable.

Rosenbaum and colleagues summed up the distinction as follows:[163]

Management implies looking at the child's day from a 24-hour perspective and ensuring that all aspects of their life are being given appropriate attention and intervention, hence the need to integrate therapy into the total management package and to appreciate the contribution of the many team members. We provide treatment to achieve management in order to enhance function and life quality.

The overall goal of management is to help the individual with spastic diplegia reach their true potential—to promote their self-confidence and independence to the greatest possible extent. This is no different from the goal parents have for any of their children. However, when it comes to the young person with spastic diplegia, the family and professionals must work hard to ensure the condition does not hold them back from achieving their potential. Reflecting the International Classification of Functioning, Disability and Health (ICF) model addressed in section 1.8, the aim of management is to promote optimal participation in daily life by enhancing activities and minimizing problems with body functions and structure. At the same time, environmental and personal factors are also considered.

This chapter examines what good management and treatment look like. It addresses management and treatment to age 20, and Chapter 4 then addresses spastic diplegia in adulthood. This age cutoff is appropriate for a couple of reasons:

- Growth is an important factor in spastic diplegia. As we saw in the growth charts in Chapter 2, growth is generally complete by age 20.
- Around age 18 to 20, health services in most countries transition from pediatric to adult. Sadly, health services for adults with CP are generally much less developed than those for children.

USEFUL WEB RESOURCES

What does best practice look like?

"Would you tell me, please, which way I ought to go from here?"
"That depends a good deal on where you want to get to," said the Cat.
"I don't much care where—" said Alice.
"Then it doesn't matter which way you go," said the Cat.

Lewis Carroll

It is important to understand what best practice in the medical care of individuals with spastic diplegia looks like. This section provides an overview of the generally accepted principles underpinning best practice in the management and treatment of spastic diplegia at the time of writing. Best practice is likely to continue to evolve over time. It currently includes:

- Family-centered care and person-centered care
- A multidisciplinary team approach
- Evidence-based medicine and shared decision-making
- Data-driven decision-making
- The importance of specialist centers
- Early intervention
- Setting goals
- Using measurement tools and measuring outcome

Family-centered care and person-centered care

When a child is diagnosed with spastic diplegia, the whole family is affected: parents, siblings, and extended family members. Family-centered care is a way of ensuring that care is planned around the whole family, not just the child with the condition.* It can be thought of as a meeting of experts who pool their knowledge to jointly develop the most appropriate plan of care for the child. The parent is the expert on their child, while the professional is the expert on the condition and its treatment. Professionals who practice family-centered care see themselves not as the sole authority but as a partner with the parent in the provision of care for the child.

Family-centered care and person-centered care are closely related. The latter evolves from the former as the child grows. In person-centered care, the individual is an active participant and decision maker in their own medical care. A few points on person-centered care:

- Person-centered care involves the professional engaging the child from an early stage in conversations. A study of factors that predict whether a child will answer questions during primary care pediatric visits found that if a doctor simply looks at a very young child when they ask a question, that child is more likely to engage in the medical process.[165]
- Person-centered care promotes the opposite of "learned helplessness," the belief that nothing one chooses to do can affect what is happening.[166] Learned helplessness can be regarded as a secondary disability.
- One study found that having learned how to take personal responsibility for personal health during childhood was significantly associated with regular physical activity in adults with CP.[167]

---

* Family-centered care is also termed "family-centered service." CanChild defines family-centered care as being "made up of a set of values, attitudes, and approaches to services for children with special needs and their families. Family-centred service recognizes that **each family is unique**; that the family is the **constant in the child's life**; and that they are the **experts on the child's abilities and needs**. The family works with service providers to make informed decisions about the services and supports the child and family receive. In family-centred service, the strengths and needs of all family members are considered."[164]

The change from family-centered care to person-centered care is gradual, and parents and medical professionals can help facilitate the shift over time.

In the early days, the child cannot speak for themselves, so the parent has to be their advocate and decision maker. A friend of mine signed all official paperwork for her young son as "Deirdre (surname), voice of John (surname)." This clearly summed up how she viewed her role.

As experts on our children, we parents must not forget to speak up on their behalf. Our child is depending on us. Here's an example: Once, a well-meaning occupational therapist suggested Tommy get a special adjustable table and chair at school to promote good posture while sitting. He was about eight or nine years old at the time. The downside was that instead of sitting at a table for two like all his peers and having the company of a friend, he was now sitting alone at a very different-looking table. He did not like it at all. Whatever the marginal gain in posture, the loss in terms of participation was simply not worth it. He stopped using it after about a year.

I advise parents to be mindful of the cost-benefit ratio of treatments. (I'm not talking about financial cost.) Remember, you are the expert on your child, and you should feel empowered to weigh the pros and cons of medical professionals' recommendations to make sure they are truly what's best for your child. Don't be afraid to offer another perspective (even if you only realize it after the fact, as I did in the example above). Trust your judgment.

A multidisciplinary team approach

A multidisciplinary team approach means the individual is being treated by medical professionals from several disciplines working together as a team, although each stays within their own professional boundaries. Optimal treatment for individuals with CP may include physical therapy (PT); occupational therapy (OT); speech and language pathology (SLP), also termed "speech and language therapy" (SLT); nursing; orthotics; pediatrics; neurology; neurosurgery; orthopedic surgery; physical medicine and rehabilitation (PM&R), also termed "physiatry"; and more.*

A more detailed explanation of the role of the team members is included in *Cerebral Palsy Road Map: What to Expect as Your Child Grows*[168] (included in **Useful web resources**).

I came across a booklet on type 2 diabetes that outlined the members of the diabetes care team. The very first answer to the question "Who is in your diabetes team?" was "You, the person with diabetes, are the most vital member of the team."

The same can be said of CP. You, the parent—and, later in life, the person with the condition—are the most vital member of the team. The person with the condition "owns" it: they can seek the best help available, but at the end of the day they still own their condition. (And in the early days, the parent owns the condition on behalf of the young child.)

To use a sporting analogy, the success of the multidisciplinary team depends on the members playing as a team, not as individuals skilled in their own positions.

Evidence-based medicine and shared decision-making

Evidence-based medicine (or evidence-based practice) is "the conscientious, explicit, and judicious use of current best evidence in making decisions about the care of individual patients."[169] It combines the best available external clinical evidence from research with the clinical expertise of the professional.[169] Family priorities and preferences are

---

* The role of PT, OT, and SLP is explained in section 3.4. **Orthotics** is concerned with the design, manufacture, and management of orthoses, devices designed to hold specific body parts in position to modify their structure and/or function. **Pediatrics** deals with children and their medical conditions. **Neurology** deals with disorders of the nervous system. **Neurosurgery** involves surgical management of disorders of the nervous system. **Orthopedic surgery** involves surgical management of disorders affecting the musculoskeletal system: the muscles, bones, joints, and their related structures. PM&R aims to enhance and restore functional ability and quality of life among those with physical disabilities.

also considered.[170] Since clinical expertise can vary, it is important to know that recommendations made in this book may be different at other hospitals and treatment centers.

Best practice management of CP is by a multidisciplinary team that is skilled in this condition and that engages with the family in a shared decision-making model. Shared decision-making is a process in which the family is actively involved in making the medical decisions. It incorporates the principles of evidence-based medicine.[171]

Unfortunately, though evidence-based practice is the goal, several authors in the field of CP have noted that there is a long way to go to achieve it.[172,173] The translation of research into clinical practice can be slow: this applies to all medical fields, not just CP. It has been found that it takes an average of 17 years for research evidence to reach clinical practice.[174] For example, the GMFCS was first published in 1997, but a 2015 published survey of 283 pediatric physical therapists found that fewer than half used the GMFCS consistently,[175] and a 2018 study found that fewer than half of 303 caregivers knew their child's GMFCS level.[176]

Implementation science is an emerging field of health care science that focuses on bridging the gap between research and its effective implementation in clinical practice. Factors that influence successful implementation include organizational behavior, clinician behavior, and patient preferences. An example is the successful implementation of the guideline for early detection of CP across a network of five US high-risk infant follow-up programs.[24] Another is the development and rollout of COVID-19 vaccines.

Funding for CP research is low, which makes the choice of research conducted very important. A 2018 US initiative to set a person-centered research agenda for CP involved a collaboration among all stakeholders—including caregivers and people with CP—based on the belief that a research agenda developed collaboratively would be more useful to the entire community than one developed by professionals alone. It was built around the concept of "nothing about us without us."*[177]

Data-driven decision-making

Best practice demands decision-making be data-driven. (This can also be called "data-informed decision-making.") For example, in orthopedic surgical decision-making in CP (e.g., for single-event multilevel surgery, or SEMLS, addressed in section 3.8), data is drawn from multiple sources, including:

- The individual's history
- Functional outcome measures and self-reported outcome measures
- Physical examination
- Imaging
- Gait analysis†
- Examination under anesthesia

The skilled evaluation of multiple sources of data is essential for good decision-making.

The importance of specialist centers

Specialist centers, also known as centers of excellence, are on the rise in many areas of medicine across the developed world. Consider, for example, specialist centers for breast cancer. Research has shown that outcomes in breast cancer treatment improve with the number of breast cancer cases a particular center has treated (this is known as centralization).[178] The annual number of operations per center and per surgeon (specialization) is also important, and the multidisciplinary team is of paramount importance.[178]

---

* Sixteen top research priorities were identified. Leading themes included the comparative effectiveness of interventions, physical activity, and understanding aging. It also highlighted the need to focus on longitudinal research that includes outcomes related to participation and quality of life.

† A measurement tool used to evaluate gait. Within gait analysis, multiple variables are evaluated using different measurement tools (see section 3.8).

A specialist center for the treatment of individuals with CP:

- Has a multidisciplinary team that includes the specialties described earlier
- Treats a high volume of patients with CP on a routine or daily basis
- Provides the full range of evidence-based treatment options, allowing the most suitable ones to be chosen for each child
- Conducts research and publishes in peer-reviewed journals
- Ideally, offers a lifetime of care; CP is not just a "children's condition"

Unless you're lucky enough to live near such a center, visiting one will likely involve travel and expense. I advise you to seek out the best specialist center in your area (the criteria listed above may be useful) and have your child reviewed there as early as possible. This doesn't mean all services have to be delivered by the specialist center. A specialist center will work with your child's local care team, but you should be able to visit it at critical times.

Early intervention

Early intervention is essential in the management of CP. Early intervention is usually from birth to age three in the US[179] and may continue beyond that age elsewhere. We have already seen that:

- Early diagnosis is necessary for early intervention.
- Early intervention offers the best opportunity to tap into neuroplasticity.
- Early intervention is important for minimizing the secondary problems as the child grows. Remember, growth is most vigorous in the first three years of life.

Though the emphasis with intervention is on early implementation, intervention continues to be required during childhood, adolescence, and adulthood.

Setting goals

Treatment goals should be collaboratively agreed upon by the child, parent, and professional as part of family-centered care and shared decision-making. The achievement of goals should be evaluated after treatment. One widely used goal-directed system used in rehabilitation is known as SMART, a system applied in many industries in areas like project management and employee performance. It is also used in personal development.

The SMART system goals are designed to be Specific, Measurable, Achievable, Relevant, and Time-bound:[180]

- **Specific** and **Measurable:** Goals that are specific and measurable should contain five elements:
  - Who
  - Will do what
  - Under what conditions
  - How well
  - By when
- **Achievable:** Goals should match the child's prognosis and be attainable.
- **Relevant:** Goals should hold meaning for the child and family. Goals should be functional; that is, not solely based on impairment (problems with body functions and structure).
- **Time-bound:** Goals must have a specific date for achievement.*

The following are some examples of SMART goals:

- James will pull to stand with furniture support in order to participate in play activities (e.g., a train table) within three months.
- Kleo will creep 30 feet (9 meters) independently in order to move between rooms of her home within three months.
- Quinn will maintain tailor sitting independently while using both hands for play for 10 minutes in order to participate in play activities within her home within six weeks.

---

* Typically, a goal would include a specific date for achievement, rather than the less specific "within three months."

- Athena will use her posterior (reverse) walker to walk 300 feet (91 meters) over the sidewalk in order to access the playground at recess within three months.
- Jack will ascend and descend 13 stairs with one rail and minimal assistance (steadying assistance of a parent) in order to access the bedroom on the upper level of his home within one month.

Research has shown that:

- Therapies that focus on achieving functional goals in everyday life result in measurable improvements in gross motor skills compared to therapies that are not goal-directed.[181]
- The development of fewer and more meaningful goals is imperative for adherence, improved outcomes, and greater individual and family satisfaction.[182]
- Children can be trusted to identify their own goals, thereby influencing their involvement in their own treatment programs. If the child creates their own goal, they will likely be more motivated to achieve it. Children's self-identified goals were found to be as achievable as parent-identified goals and remained stable over time (i.e., achievements were maintained).[183]
- A family-centered approach to intervention has been shown to improve motivation and outcome.[184]

A number of tools are available to incorporate family goals. Some of the more common ones are the Canadian Occupational Performance Measure (COPM),[185] the Goal Attainment Scale,[186] and the Gait Outcomes Assessment List (GOAL).[187,188,189,190]

Using measurement tools and measuring outcome

Many variables can be measured, including height, walking speed, and walking ability. Some variables can be measured using equipment, others by parent or self-report (e.g., by completing a questionnaire). A tape measure, timed walk test, gait analysis, the Gillette Functional

Assessment Questionnaire (FAQ),* and the GOAL are all examples of measurement tools used to measure these variables. A measurement can be taken at any point in time to establish a person's status at that point in time.

An outcome is defined as a result or an effect; thus, "measuring outcome" means measuring a result or an effect. If a person's walking speed is measured before a treatment such as orthopedic surgery and then again afterward, the effect or result—the outcome—of the surgery on the person's walking speed can be evaluated.

Variables used to measure outcome can be classified as technical, functional, or by patient/parent satisfaction. For example, orthopedic surgery is commonly evaluated using many technical variables (joint ROM, gait deviations, energy consumed in walking) as well as functional variables (gross motor function, walking ability). Each variable provides different but complementary information. Variables can be measured in each domain of the ICF (body functions and structure, activity, and participation). A range of variables covering different domains of the ICF provides the most comprehensive evaluation of outcome. Appendix 1 (online) includes more information on measurement tools.

We parents want the very best for our children with spastic diplegia. We understand that it is a lifelong condition and that there is currently no cure. Our children deserve the best management and treatment to ensure the effects of their condition are no more burdensome than they absolutely need to be. We want its management to be limited only by medical science.

The reality, however, is that the quality and standard of available services varies greatly between countries, and even within a country. Some areas have much better services than others. Management of a child's

---

* The Gillette FAQ includes a family report 10-level walking scale. It asks the individual/family to rate the individual's typical walking ability with their usual mobility aids. The scale covers a range of walking ability from level 1 ("Cannot take any steps at all") to level 10 ("Walks, runs, and climbs on level and uneven terrain and does stairs without difficulty or assistance. Is typically able to keep up with peers").

(or adolescent's or adult's) condition should not be limited by zip or postal code.

Many professionals may themselves wish they could provide more and better services to people with CP. They, too, may recognize gaps in their service provision. Rosenbaum and Rosenbloom noted that both parents and professionals need to be aware of what effective services look like and lobby health policy-makers in unison to improve services.[8] I agree: we parents need to know what good management and treatment looks like, and if the services in our community or country do not measure up, we need to lobby to effect change, even if doing so is challenging. Otherwise, our children, adolescents, and adults with CP are the ones who lose out.

Overall management philosophy

When there is no turning back, then we should concern ourselves only with the best way of going forward.

Paulo Coelho

The definition of CP describes it first as a disorder of the development of movement and posture, causing activity limitation that is often accompanied by disturbances of sensation, perception, cognition, communication, and behavior, by epilepsy, and by secondary musculoskeletal problems.[2] While a lot of attention is given to development of movement and posture and secondary musculoskeletal problems, for some individuals with spastic diplegia, difficulties with communication or learning may pose bigger barriers to participation. In section 2.1, we saw that children with spastic diplegia:

- Have problems with gross motor function; 63 percent are functioning at GMFCS levels I and II and 23 percent at GMFCS levels III
- Have problems with fine motor ability; however, 76 percent are functioning at MACS levels I and II

We saw that across all GMFCS levels, children age five with spastic diplegia had some level of problem with speech (48 percent), hearing (10 percent), vision (30 percent), intellectual status (39 percent), and epilepsy (14 percent).[80] Problems with, for example, speech, language, and cognition, if present, may be more challenging for the individual with spastic diplegia than their lower limb functional limitations.

The following are some pointers in the overall management of spastic diplegia in childhood and adolescence:

- CP-specific early interventions are designed to:[21]
  - Optimize motor, cognition, and communication skills using interventions that promote learning and neuroplasticity
  - Prevent secondary impairments and minimize complications that worsen function or interfere with learning (e.g., monitor hips, control epilepsy, take care of sleeping, feeding)
  - Promote parent or caregiver coping and mental health
- Morgan and colleagues published an International Clinical Practice Guideline for early intervention for children age 0 to 2 with or at high risk of CP.[30] They followed this with another guideline in 2023 for children in the first year of life, which helps decide what kind of motor intervention to choose from based on the motor problem.[34] Earlier, Novak and colleagues summarized the state of the evidence as of 2019 for interventions for children with CP. They used a traffic light system:[14]
  - Green means go because high-quality evidence indicates the effectiveness of that intervention.
  - Red means stop because high-quality evidence indicates the ineffectiveness or harm from that intervention.
  - Yellow means measure clinical outcome (i.e., measure the effect of the intervention on the individual) because the evidence either does not exist or is yet unclear on the benefit of the intervention.

  The above guidelines help therapists support families, and links to them are included in **Useful web resources.**

- Primary, secondary, and tertiary problems are addressed in sections 2.6. to 2.8. Other than high tone and to a limited extent weakness, the primary problems (the neurological problems) are difficult to treat. The secondary problems (the growth problems) can often be treated, and treatment for the tertiary problems (coping responses or compensations) is generally not necessary.

- Monitoring musculoskeletal development is a constant throughout childhood and adolescence. It includes, for example, physical examination, X-rays, and gait analysis.
- Treatment of musculoskeletal concerns in spastic diplegia generally begins at diagnosis with physical and occupational therapies. Over time, orthoses and casting may be added, and tone reduction* may be considered as well. Different treatments, when used together, can amplify the effect of individual treatments; for example, attending therapies to achieve a new functional goal following botulinum neurotoxin A (BoNT-A) injections.† The saying, "The whole is greater than the sum of its parts" applies.
- While the lower limbs are much more affected in spastic diplegia than the upper limbs, which frequently show only fine motor impairment, we have included Appendix 2 (online) on managing upper limb problems, for those whose upper limbs are affected. Individuals with spastic diplegia, GMFCS levels I to III generally do not need tone reduction or orthopedic surgery for upper limb problems.
- Hip surveillance and spine surveillance are structured approaches to monitoring the development of the hips and spine respectively in individuals with CP and should start early in life:
  - The risk of hip displacement for children with CP at GMFCS level I is the same as typically developing children, but it is 15 percent for those at GMFCS level II and 41 percent for those at GMFCS level III.[127,128]
  - The AACPDM (American Academy for Cerebral Palsy and Developmental Medicine) has developed a care pathway to monitor hip development in children and adolescents with CP (included in **Useful web resources**). It includes recommendations for the timing of clinical examination and X-rays.

---

* An **orthosis** (also termed "brace" or "splint") is a device designed to hold specific body parts in position in order to modify their structure and/or function. **Casting** consists of applying a plaster of paris or a fiberglass cast; for example, a below-knee cast to stretch the tight gastrocnemius and/or soleus muscles (calf muscles) to hold the muscle in a position of maximum stretch. **Tone reduction** is addressed in detail in section 3.7.

† BoNT-A is a tone-reducing medication that is injected directly into the muscle.

- ○ Formal hip surveillance programs for children and adolescents with CP have been implemented in a number of countries, including Australia and Sweden.[3,191]
- ○ Unlike hip surveillance, no formal guidelines exist for spine surveillance at this time. However, we saw in Chapter 2 that for individuals at GMFCS levels I to III, scoliosis curves (Cobb angle greater than 10 degrees) are uncommon, generally small, mostly nonprogressive, and with minimal or no symptoms.[136] However, Willoughby and colleagues recommend that small curves be monitored.[136] Management of scoliosis for individuals with spastic diplegia is included in Appendix 3 (online).
- Despite best efforts, and for the reasons described in Chapter 2, the development of some muscle and bone problems is largely inevitable in individuals with spastic diplegia. Depending on the degree to which they impact function and participation, orthopedic surgery may be recommended. Single-event multilevel surgery (SEMLS)—a single operation to address all muscle and bone problems at once—is often used. An intensive period of rehabilitation can help achieve a higher level of function following surgery. Orthopedic surgery is addressed in section 3.8.
  - ○ Unpublished data from Gillette Children's indicate that approximately 70 percent of children with spastic diplegia require lower limb SEMLS. SEMLS for the lower limb is best carried out between the ages of 6 and 12.[192]
  - ○ SEMLS does not alter the primary problems of CP, and a gradual recurrence of some muscle and bone problems may occur in a proportion of individuals post-SEMLS.
- Overall, minimizing the amount of orthopedic surgery needed remains an important goal. Because growth is a major factor in musculoskeletal care, once growth ceases at around age 20, a certain stabilization of the condition occurs. No treatment should ever be viewed as an end point. All treatments are aids in the pursuit of the overall goal of getting to skeletal maturity (i.e., adulthood) with the fewest possible problems.
- It is also worth noting that no treatment (with today's treatments) will give full function to the affected limbs.

Finally, the home program (addressed in section 3.4) is a constant in the life of the child and adolescent with spastic diplegia.

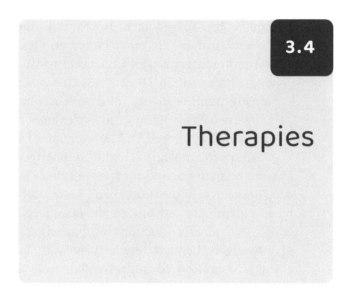

Therapies

The nice thing about teamwork is that you
always have others on your side.

Margaret Carty

Many children with spastic diplegia attend physical therapy, occupational therapy, and/or speech and language pathology at various points during their development. Therapy is defined by Rosenbaum and colleagues as:

> *A process of helping a family (and a child) to learn ways for a child to function optimally in their many environments. It … involves using the therapist's expertise to explore ways that will enable the child and the family to live as fully and functionally as possible.*[163]

Obviously, this definition extends to the adolescent and adult with CP as well. Improvement in function should be the primary goal of therapy.

This section covers:

- **Physical therapy**
- **Occupational therapy**
- **Speech and language pathology**[*]
- **Delivery of therapy services**
- **Getting the most out of appointments**

Physical therapy

Physical therapists provide services that develop, maintain, and restore a person's maximum movement and functional ability.[193] Physical therapists have different titles in different countries: in many countries they are called physiotherapists. In this book, we use the terms "physical therapist" and "physical therapy."[†]

Services that pediatric physical therapists provide for children and adolescents with CP may include:[170]

- Developmental activities
- Movement and mobility
- Strengthening
- Motor learning
- Balance and coordination
- Recreation, play, and leisure
- Daily care activities and routines
- Equipment design, making, and fitting
- Tone management
- Assistive technology (including orthoses)
- Posture, positioning, and lifting

---

[*] There are other types of therapy offered by specialists: for example, play therapists, music therapists, and recreational therapists. A recreational therapist is qualified to provide recreational therapy services in the US and Canada. There may be an equivalent professional in other countries.

[†] In Ireland, the terms "physical therapist" and "physiotherapist" are not interchangeable. There, a "physical therapist" is someone trained specifically in the manual treatment of soft tissues, mostly massage.

Physical therapists work as part of the multidisciplinary team taking care of the child or adolescent.

Though physical therapists may select treatments designed to improve functional activities, the treatments themselves are often not strictly functional activities. For example, a child's goal may be to be able to get up from the floor without holding on to anything for support. During the evaluation, the physical therapist may identify limited ankle range of motion (ROM) and weak hip and knee extensors on the affected side as the underlying problems preventing the child from meeting their goal. As a result, the physical therapist might include casting (to address the limited ROM) and isolated strengthening exercises (to address the weak extensors) on the affected side in the plan of care for that child with spastic diplegia. These treatments address the underlying problems, but they themselves are not functional activities. However, as the underlying problems are reduced, the treatment will shift to *task-specific functional activities*. In this example, the child begins to practice moving from the floor to standing.

Another example is if the child's physical therapy (PT) goal is to walk more independently, then the therapy might primarily involve walking and the many activities that form the building blocks for walking.

Thus, treatments are often task-specific functional activities. Research supports task-specific training (green light) for improved gross motor function.[14]

We now address some elements of PT in more detail.

a) Strengthening

Lack of muscle strength is one of the primary problems, but muscle strength is further affected by the development of the secondary problems (abnormal muscle growth and bone development). We saw in Chapter 2 that muscle strength was reduced in children with spastic diplegia.[111,194] Historically, strengthening was frowned upon because it was thought to increase spasticity. However it now is known to increase the force-producing capability, not the spasticity, of the muscle,[195] and therefore strengthening is recommended.

The physical therapist can determine which strengthening exercises are appropriate for the child at their developmental stage. Muscles can be strengthened in different positions. Strengthening may be functional, like moving into sitting from standing, or from standing to sitting, or stair climbing.

In addition to doing focused muscle strengthening exercises, strengthening has to be built into normal life. For the small child, a variety of positions can provide an opportunity to strengthen the muscles during play. Often, those same positions can be used to achieve both stretch and strength. The need for strengthening also applies to the older child and adolescent.

Research supports strength training for improved lower limb strength (green light).[14]

b) Functional mobility and gait training

Physical therapists specialize in movement, and a significant amount of PT is focused on practicing functional mobility. The physical therapist selects specific mobility activities or tasks based on the individual's age, function, as well as the family's goals.

For very young children, physical therapists emphasize practicing developmental activities such as rolling, creeping, and crawling. Later, they may emphasize moving from one position to another such as moving in and out of standing positions or moving with support (e.g., cruising—when the child walks alongside a sofa while holding on for support). Depending on the child's function and environmental demands, physical therapists may teach children to use different movements* or

---

* For example, nonreciprocal rather than reciprocal crawling. Reciprocal crawling involves coordinated movements of opposite hands and knees to move forward; nonreciprocal crawling refers to any form of movement (e.g., using a single hand to drag themselves forward without coordinating both sides of the body).

recommend the use of orthoses or mobility aids* to maximize the child's independence.

For older children, adolescents, and adults, functional mobility includes how a person moves in and out of bed, transfers (stands up and sits down or moves from chair to chair) and moves around in their environment (walking or using a wheelchair).

Another area of focus is gait training, an intervention to work on developing or improving walking skills. As with other aspects of functional mobility, physical therapists may recommend the use of orthoses or mobility aids to maximize the child's independence. Physical therapists (in collaboration with the multidisciplinary team) are a great source of guidance on mobility aids and orthoses to use in daily life.

Gait training is often a progression. It may initially require more assistance and more-supportive mobility aids but progress to less assistance and less-supportive mobility aids. It may also progress to increasing distances and walking in more challenging environments. Conversely, following surgery or based on environmental demands (e.g., moving between classes on a large high school or college campus), more-supportive mobility aids and orthoses might be recommended to reduce fatigue, pain, and/or falls, which speaks to the competing goals: there is a balance to be struck between independent walking and using mobility aids and orthoses; the latter may allow the person to participate more fully in everyday life.

Specific gait training interventions used during therapy may include treadmill training, body weight support treadmill training, and various forms of assisted and even robotic training. Using a treadmill can

---

* Mobility aids (also termed "assistive mobility devices," "assistive devices," "walking aids," and "gait aids") vary in the level of support they provide. Here they are listed in order of least to most support:
  • Canes (walking sticks)
  • Crutches
  • Reverse walker
  • Gait trainer (a device that is more supportive than a walker but less supportive than a wheelchair).
  • Wheelchair
Canes may be single or triple-pronged (three-point). Triple-pronged canes provide more support if the person has balance issues. There are also quadruple-pronged (four-point) canes for even greater support. One or two canes or crutches may be used. Wheelchairs may be self-propelled or power-assisted.

be helpful to focus on increased speed or symmetry. Harnesses can be used to provide body weight support or for safety when walking on the floor or treadmill. Lower limb robotics is a growing aspect of CP therapy.[196] For example, robotic-assisted training may involve using an exoskeleton* to provide some assistance to move the legs while walking. The emphasis during these interventions is on practicing a high number of repetitions or steps, providing the opportunity to learn from errors, decreasing support, and getting practice in a variety of environments.

Research supports treadmill training for improved walking speed, endurance, and gross motor function (green light) and improved weight-bearing (yellow light).[14]

c) Electrical stimulation

Neuromuscular electrical stimulation (NMES), also simply termed "electrical stimulation" (ES), is a treatment (and not a task-specific functional activity) that involves the electrical stimulation of nerves to produce a muscle contraction. Functional electrical stimulation (FES), a subtype of NMES, involves electrical stimulation that produces a contraction to obtain a functionally useful movement. Electrodes are placed on the muscle and a device transmits the electrical current through a wired or wireless connection.

Electrical stimulation is usually used in combination with functional activities and for muscle strengthening. It may also be used during gait training (e.g., to stimulate the ankle dorsiflexor during swing phase).

Research supports electrical stimulation for improved walking and strength (yellow light).[14]

d) Stretching

Stretching is not a task-specific functional activity, but it is still important in spastic diplegia; it helps to improve or maintain joint ROM and alignment.

---

* A wearable robotic device designed to help with walking by providing external support to the wearer's lower limbs.

The physical therapist can provide guidance, but stretching must be built into the activities of normal life. We saw in Chapter 2 that two to four hours of stretching per day is required for normal muscle growth, and the typically developing child gets this amount of stretch during the day when they get up and start to move about, run, and play using a normal movement pattern. We also saw that lack of muscle growth leads to contractures in people with spastic diplegia.

Stretching is required throughout growth for the young child, the older child, and the adolescent with spastic diplegia. How this stretching is achieved may vary over the years, but the need for it remains constant. There are also critical periods when stretching is especially important during the periods of most rapid growth: the first three years and the adolescent growth spurt.

Though we refer to stretching muscles, what is actually being stretched is the muscle, the tendon, and all the tissues that surround them called the muscle-tendon unit (MTU) and the associated joint. Muscles responsible for the movements (left column of Table 2.4.1) are in particular need of stretching because they are affected by spasticity. It is worth becoming familiar with these.

The methods used for stretching depend on a number of factors, including level of spasticity, muscle tightness, age, and developmental stage.

Traditionally, stretching was done by performing slow *passive* stretching[*] of spastic muscles. However, due to weak evidence supporting the efficacy of passive stretching, greater emphasis is now placed on other, active methods of achieving muscle stretch.[197] Novak and colleagues concur that passive stretching in isolation appears to be ineffective and do not recommend it since effective substitutes exist.[14] While passive stretching is sometimes still needed, it should not be the only method used.

The following describes different methods of stretching (any number of which may be used simultaneously).

---

[*] When another person stretches an individual's muscle.

i) Positioning

A variety of positions can be used throughout the day to achieve sustained muscle stretching to promote muscle growth. It is important that the child or adolescent get a variety of positions throughout the day and not spend too much time in one. They may have favorite positions, but it is important to vary them. For the small child, moving between positions may require parental support.

"W-sitting" is the term used to describe the sitting position in which the child's bottom is on the floor while their legs are out to each side. Looking from the top, the legs form a "W" shape. (See Figure 3.4.1.) Children with spastic diplegia like W-sitting because it is a stable position, requires less balance, and leaves the hands free for play. The problem with W-sitting is that it may cause a loss of hip external rotation, which interrupts the typical process of bone remodeling. The child also misses out on functional opportunities to develop balance reactions. While W-sitting was traditionally not recommended, it is now thought to be somewhat acceptable provided the child gets plenty of time in other positions to balance out the less ideal elements of W-sitting.

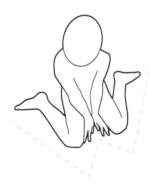

Figure 3.4.1 Child W-sitting.

For older children and adolescents with spastic diplegia, it is also very important to not spend prolonged time in one position, usually sitting—a particular challenge given the not uncommon overuse of electronic devices.

Appendix 4 (online) includes information on various positions, including long sitting, side sitting, tailor sitting, prone positioning, and standing. It is important to look for a lot of opportunities during the day to incorporate different positioning—for example, while playing, reading, watching TV, or using electronic devices.

ii) Orthoses

An orthosis (also termed "brace" or "splint") is a device designed to hold specific body parts in position in order to modify their structure and/or function. One of the goals of orthoses is to achieve muscle stretch for a longer duration.

Night splints, such as ankle-foot orthoses (AFOs), which cover the ankle joint and foot, plus knee immobilizers,* may also be used to achieve stretching at night. Wearing an AFO plus a knee immobilizer allows stretching of the calf muscles (both the one-joint soleus and the two-joint gastrocnemius; see Table 2.4.1). Night splints are worn to tolerance during sleep. Wearing one knee immobilizer each night and alternating between right and left may help if wearing both at once is too much.

Orthoses are discussed in section 3.6.

iii) Casting

Casting consists of applying a plaster of paris or a fiberglass cast; for example a below-knee cast to stretch the tight gastrocnemius and/or soleus muscles (calf muscles) to hold the muscle in a position of maximum stretch. Fiberglass casts are lighter and allow weight-bearing. Serial casting is the application, removal, and reapplication of stretching casts (e.g., weekly, for several weeks, typically three to six weeks) to gain ROM with each subsequent casting until the desired ROM is achieved.

iv) Active movement

Active movement is exactly what it sounds like. The child or adolescent needs to get plenty of active movement through the entire ROM of the joints. They can remove orthoses if they are hindering doing a task and replace them during downtime for a prolonged muscle stretch. This

---

* A knee immobilizer consists of a soft knee wrap, rigid aluminum struts, and straps to adjust the fit. As the name suggests, it prevents the knee from moving.

gives them a combination of active movement that may not be in the "best" position, and static stretch in the ideal position.

The approach used in physical therapy and many of the treatments are also used in occupational therapy, addressed next.

> Once parents understand the key muscles that need stretching and/ or strengthening, they can look for opportunities to incorporate these activities into the child's play. For example, the hip adductors (the inner thigh muscles) are often tight, while the hip abductors (the outer thigh muscles) are often weak. One can make a game of side walking on a playground or around the perimeter of the shallow end of a swimming pool. These can be fun ways for the young child to stretch the adductors and strengthen the abductors in everyday life.

Occupational therapy

Occupational therapists use everyday activities (occupations) to promote health, well-being, and independence throughout an individual's life.[198] They work with children and adolescents to build confidence and independence through:

- Completing meaningful tasks to maximize independent movement, strength, and coordination
- Compensating or modifying activities or the environment to enable successful task completion
- Recommending or providing equipment (e.g., orthoses, wheelchairs, bathing equipment) and/or technology that can increase independence when performing activities

Basically, the above are in priority order: 1) try to build or remediate skill, 2) compensate or modify task to meet the individual's skill, 3) use equipment to support function.

Areas covered in occupational therapy (OT) include, but are not limited to:

- Daily living skills such as dressing, feeding, grooming, and bathing

- Fine motor skills such as writing, using scissors, and manipulating toys
- Cognitive skills such as sticking to a schedule, learning to play a new game, and following step-by-step directions
- Visual motor skills and visual perceptual skills such as using eye movement to explore and interact with the environment
- Participation in the day-to-day activities that motivate the person, such as play, sport, crafts, and vocational skills
- Range of motion, strengthening, and coordination of postural muscles and arms for functional tasks

Occupational therapists can be especially important as the child grows, when daily activities and independent living skills become more demanding and potentially more difficult to complete.

Speech and language pathology

Speech and language pathology (SLP) is also known as speech and language therapy (SLT). Speech-language pathologists/therapists work with children, young people, and adults to support speech, language, and communication needs as well as feeding and swallowing difficulties. The following are explanations of terms:

- **Speech** refers to saying sounds accurately and in the right places in words. Speech is a motor task.
- **Language** refers to the words and symbols we use, and how we use them for communication. Language is a cognitive task.*
- **Receptive language** refers to understanding information from sounds, words, symbols, signs, gestures, and/or movements.
- **Expressive language** refers to the ability to communicate thoughts, wants, needs, and/or feelings through words, gestures, signs, and/or symbols.
- **Communication** occurs when a sender transmits a message, and a receiver understands the message. Communication includes speech, gestures, behaviors, eye gaze, facial expressions, and augmentative and alternative communication (AAC).[62]

---

* Cognition is the mental action of acquiring knowledge and understanding through thought, experience, and the senses.

Speech-language pathologists assess speech, language, and cognitive skills to determine how to improve communication. The child and adolescent may receive SLP at school, in an outpatient clinic, or both. Just as there is overlap between PT and OT, there is overlap between OT and SLP. The speech-language pathologist will work with parents, teachers, and others to identify strategies that encourage and improve the child's communication at home, in school, and with friends, as well as during activities to help develop speech and language skills.

SLP may be done individually or in a group. The following are areas of focus:

- **Language skills** allow a child to communicate in their environment, which encourages the development of cognitive skills. A speech-language pathologist will work on cognitive development by improving language comprehension; building vocabulary; and teaching how to use words, gestures, and pictures to express thoughts, ideas, and feelings, and to know how to answer questions. Language comprehension is needed to be able to follow directions, understand the meaning of words, and understand how words go together.
- **Expressive language** allows a person to ask for what they want and need, to comment or provide information, to ask questions or ask for clarification if they don't understand, to request attention when needed, and to express feelings.
- **Oral motor skills** improve secretion management (drooling, aspiration of secretions*), which helps improve the ability to move and break down food in preparation for swallowing, for speech production, and for breathing safely.
- **Speech production** includes being able to say individual sounds accurately, with correct placement of the lips, tongue, and mouth shape, paired with adequate breath support and control of the breath stream. It also includes making the vocal folds (voice box) vibrate for some sounds and not for others. Speech production also can include sequencing of these sounds to make words, and sequencing of more than one word to make a sentence that is understood by others.

---

* Drooling is excess saliva dropping uncontrollably from the mouth. Aspiration is food or liquid entering the airway or lungs instead of the esophagus.

- **Social communication** includes how to take turns; how to partner with others to exchange ideas, thoughts, and jokes; and how to greet others. Social communication often impacts a person's ability to make and maintain friendships.
- **Cognitive-communication skills** include memory, attention, problem-solving, and organization. Attention to the environment, to the communication and language of others, and to what is happening in the environment is very important for cognitive development. Executive function includes many cognitive-communication skills that help the individual plan and get things done.
- **Fostering independence** helps the individual advocate for and communicate their wants and needs, as well as their feelings. It helps them develop autonomy and self-agency.

Tommy had delayed language development and attended SLT at an early age. He was delayed in expressive speech; his vocabulary was very limited relative to his age. (I still have the short list of his early words.)

I remember Tommy doing his SLT homework, which began with practicing the various sounds that were problematic for him. Fast-forward to age 13 when Tommy won a Best Overall Communicator award at a large national science competition for best explanation/discussion of a project in conversation with judges. It was a very sweet moment. (His project was called "What are the issues faced by children with CP in mainstream education?") Indeed, language would become very important for Tommy. During his teenage years, he wrote an award-winning blog. After completing secondary (high) school in Ireland, Tommy attended New York University and graduated cum laude in 2017 with a degree in journalism and won the David James Burrell Prize for media criticism. Those who meet Tommy as an adult would be surprised to learn of his delayed speech and language development.

His early SLT was also very important because his therapist referred him for complete review by the multidisciplinary team at the Central Remedial Clinic (CRC) in Dublin. That started our long association with the clinic.

Delivery of therapy services

Given that the delivery of therapy services is so variable, only some broad points are addressed here. Having a lifelong condition such as spastic diplegia does not mean a person will need lifelong, nonstop PT (or other therapies) or, as it is sometimes referred to, the "once a week for life" model.

Guidelines have been developed for determining the frequency of PT and OT services in a pediatric medical setting.[199] The guidelines are based on:

- The child's ability to benefit from and participate in therapy
- The parent's ability to participate in therapy sessions and follow through with activities at home
- The family's decision related to available resources (e.g., time commitment, financial resources)

Four levels of frequency of therapy are identified in the guidelines:[199]

- **Intensive:** More than three times per week—for children who are in an extremely critical period for acquiring a skill or are regressing.
- **Weekly/bimonthly:** One to two times a week to every other week—for children who need frequent therapy and are making continuous progress toward their goals.
- **Periodic:** Once a month or less—best suited to children whose rates of progress are very slow but who require the skilled services of a therapist to periodically assess a home program and adapt it.
- **Consultative:** As needed—best suited for children who have been discharged from therapy but who benefit from intermittent evaluation by a therapist.

The episodes of care (EOC) model is used for service delivery. An EOC is a period of therapy at the recommended frequency, such as listed above, followed by a therapy break. Ideally, after an EOC, the child generalizes the skills gained in therapy at home, in school, and in the community. For each EOC, the family and therapist work together to draw up goals, typically no more than two long-term and four short-term goals. Note that referring to "therapy breaks" might sound like getting therapy is the normal state of affairs for a person with CP, but living life, not receiving therapy, should be considered the normal state of affairs.

Figure 3.4.2 shows periods when different therapies may be used, interspersed with breaks in therapy, during childhood and adolescence.[200]

In addition to having formal goals, it is very important that therapists use objective measurement tools to evaluate whether therapy goals have been met. The home program, which includes practicing what the child has learned in therapy at home and incorporating it into normal life, is addressed in section 3.5.

The following are included in **Useful web resources:**

- Cincinnati Children's *Guidelines for Determining Frequency of Therapy* information leaflet for families
- Gillette Children's *Rehabilitation Therapies Episodes of Care in Childhood and Adolescence* information leaflet for families

Getting the most out of appointments

Life with a diagnosis of spastic diplegia involves many appointments, particularly in the early years. During the COVID pandemic, virtual appointments became a feature of health care delivery, and a mixture of in-person and virtual care delivery has remained in place since.

Try to ensure you are getting as much as possible from these appointments. It is useful to go with a written list of questions and to take notes after each appointment, including what you learned and what is needed to be done next. While portals to access personal medical records (where they exist) have helped reduce the need for taking notes, you may still find it useful to do some note-taking.

To get the most out of appointments on a practical level, try to ensure your child is not tired or hungry. (For that matter, make sure *you* are not tired or hungry either!)

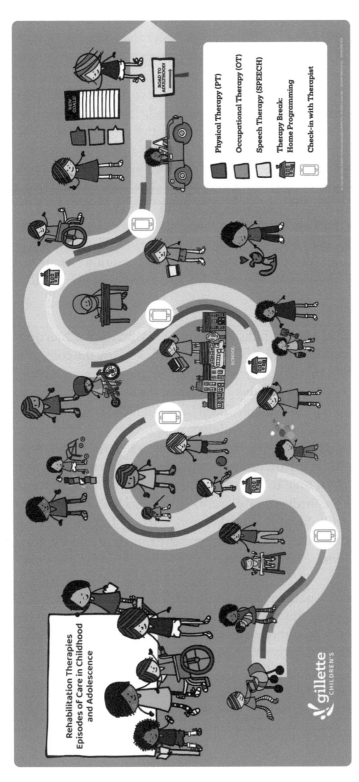

Figure 3.4.2 Episodes of care in childhood and adolescence.[200]

You know your child best, and to best support their success in therapies, you should engage with the therapy team whenever you have questions, as you might see something they do not. It is also okay to request a break or a change in activity, or to ask about the purpose of an exercise. Partner with your therapists to help optimize the care being provided. Nurture the relationship with the professionals treating your child—they are your allies. You may be angry about aspects of your child's diagnosis or treatment, but avoid putting professionals on the receiving end of any misplaced anger. The expression "Don't shoot the messenger" comes to mind. You might be dissatisfied with the range of services provided to your child, for example, but remember that frontline staff are rarely the policy-makers—indeed, they may in fact agree with you. The best management of the condition is achieved when parent and child work together in partnership with the medical professionals.

Good communication between disciplines is also vital for the functioning of the multidisciplinary team. The parent and child are the constants in this relationship; thus, the parent can help support communication between the different team members. No matter how good services are, things can go wrong: for example, a referral might be forgotten, and an appointment might not get scheduled. Supporting communication between team members is particularly important when the child is getting a large part of their care in the community but has to travel to a specialist center from time to time. The parent can play an important role in the smooth coordination of care, so it is helpful to stay organized and keep medical reports together and at hand. This coordinator role may later fall to the adolescent themselves, in time, and if their development permits.

Finally, sometimes a particular medical professional is not the right match for the family. If this occurs, be sure to communicate this and try to seek an alternative to optimize the chances of success for the child or adolescent with CP.

Spastic diplegia is managed by a multidisciplinary team. The physical therapist is likely one of the first members you will meet, and you will likely have regular contact during childhood and adolescence. Though physical therapists move jobs and change roles, your physical therapist will probably work with your family for a long time. They will get to know you and your child well.

Unless you have a health care background, raising a child with spastic diplegia involves a lot of new information. There's a lot to absorb. Therapists can be a great source of support and advice. I have very fond memories of a number of therapists who treated Tommy over the years. It truly felt like the family, not just the child, was being cared for—definitely family-centered care in practice.

As noted earlier, research supports the goal-directed/functional training approach to therapy described in this section, but there are and have been other therapy approaches. Some, but not all, have supporting evidence.

Conductive education is an example of another therapy approach. It is based on the philosophy of Professor András Pető, who founded the Pető Institute in Budapest, Hungary. It combines treatment and education into one program. The term "conductor" is used to refer to the therapist trained in conductive education. A single conductor provides the therapies we would recognize as PT, OT, and SLP/SLT. Novak and colleagues gave it a yellow light for improved gross motor skills.[14]

We used conductive education when Tommy was two to three years old. A conductor from Hungary who trained at the Pető Institute worked with Tommy for about 10 three-week blocks over a period of approximately 15 months. The program consisted of exercises and activities for three hours in the morning and one hour in the afternoon. Tommy had to put everything into practice throughout the day: the way he ate, dressed, brushed his teeth, played on the playground, etc. It was intense and tiring for a small child, but the conductor, Szilvia, had a wonderful way with him. She was very firm, but also warm and friendly.

While Tommy was undergoing conductive education, Szilvia stayed with our family. She insisted that Tommy go to bed on time each night and get up early each morning, ready to start the program at 9 a.m. When she returned to Hungary, we continued the program until her next visit.

While at that time we had not set formal goals for Tommy's conductive education, nor were we using tools to measure outcome, I can certainly say it was a successful treatment. Tommy began walking independently just after his third birthday. (I only realized while writing this book that this was earlier than predicted for him using the GMFCS.) I don't have data on how widely used this approach is today.

When we decided to try conductive education, we did so quietly. We had to: at that time, families were discharged from conventional services if they were using any other form of treatment. Nowadays I find the medical establishment is far more open, and parents can and should feel comfortable discussing other treatment options with professionals. Parents and professionals both want what's best for the child. However, I have one strong piece of advice for parents considering any alternative form of treatment: be sure there is an evidence base to support its effectiveness. (Alternative and complementary treatments are addressed in section 3.10.)

Following are several photographs from Tommy's period of conductive education. They indicate some of the progression in his learning to walk: using a ladder-back chair, parallel bars, ropes, two tripods, single stick, and independent walking.

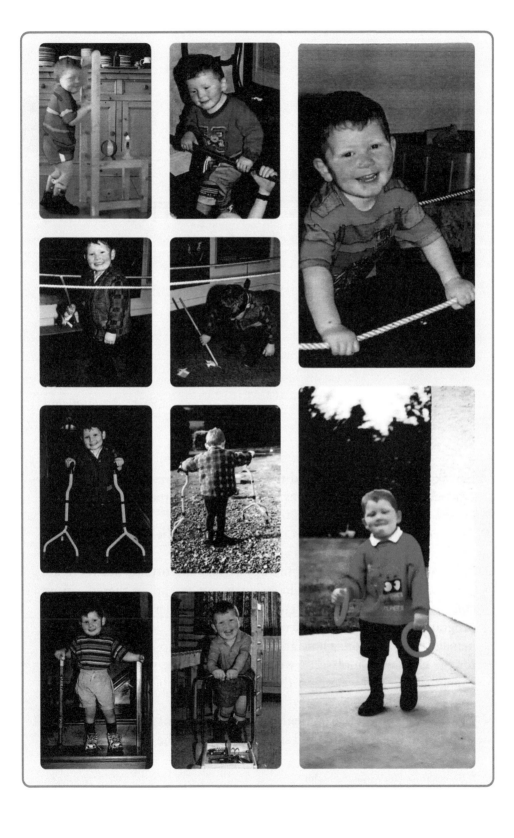

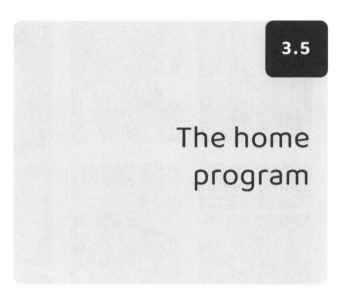

3.5

The home program

Exercise is medicine.
Susruta

Novak and colleagues defined the home program as the "therapeutic*
practice of goal-based tasks by the child, led by the parent, and supported by the therapist in the home environment."[201] In this book, we
have termed this the "homework" prescribed by therapists.

Practicing what is learned in therapy is very important, but there are
periods when the child or adolescent is not attending therapy in an
episode of care, so it makes sense to have a broader view of the home
program to include all the elements that families do at home to help
manage the condition. These are things that have to become part of life
for the child and adolescent with spastic diplegia, such as stretching,
strengthening, and wearing orthoses (when prescribed).

The term "home environment" is a collective of the actual home,
school, and wherever the child spends their time. The best people to help

---

* Recommended for reasons of health.

with the child's program are those who regularly interact with the child. In addition to parents, they may be siblings, teachers, teaching assistants, grandparents, and childcare providers. They are the optimal ones to provide developmentally appropriate opportunities. Therapists are there to teach, guide, and support.

The saying "It takes a village to raise a child" emphasizes the idea that raising a child, particularly a child with a disability, is not a task that should be shouldered by parents alone. By enlisting the support of others, parents can lighten their load and create a network of individuals who are invested in the child's well-being.

Within the broader view of the home program, it is important to never forget to have fun—one of the F-words introduced in Chapter 1. This section addresses:

- **The homework prescribed by therapists**
- **Postural management**
- **Exercise and physical activity**

The homework prescribed by therapists

The benefit of any therapy (PT, OT, SLP/SLT) is only partly gained in the therapy session itself. The real benefits come from regular practice at home. It's like learning how to play the piano: true learning does not happen during the weekly lesson but through consistent practice at home.

Families depend on therapists to prescribe evidence-based treatments. Therapists depend on the child or adolescent, with the support of the parent and their network, to get in the practice at home. This is a collaborative relationship. Much of what is learned in therapy has to become part of everyday life for the child or adolescent with spastic diplegia in order to be effective.

Working with a therapist is a partnership, and the parent and child or adolescent are partners with the therapist in the decision-making process. It is important that the parent and child or adolescent share with the therapist their goals and what may be less important to them to enable focus on what is truly valued by the team. It is recommended that you talk with your therapist and make sure you have a good understanding of the activities you'll be carrying out at home and that it is a realistic plan.

Postural management

Postural management is another constant in the life of the child and adolescent with spastic diplegia. "Posture" refers to the position in which a person holds their body while sitting, standing, or lying down. Good posture applies to everyone, not just individuals with CP.

For example, to maintain good posture, a person needs to have adequate strength in their trunk-stabilizing muscles and good balance reactions. This is why the typically developing child cannot sit independently until they are approximately six months old. Table 3.5.1 lists recommendations on good posture in sitting, standing, and sleeping.

Table 3.5.1 Good posture in sitting, standing, and sleeping

GOOD POSTURE IN:	ILLUSTRATION
Sitting • Feet flat on the floor, with hips, knees, and ankles at 90 degrees and both sides of the trunk straight and symmetrical. (If feet cannot reach the floor, something firm, such as a box or book, can be placed under them to ensure they are flat and that the 90-degree angle is achieved.) • Support provided at the sides, if necessary, to ensure the trunk is straight and symmetrical. • Arms close to the body and relaxed. • Head balanced on the neck (not tilted forward or backward).	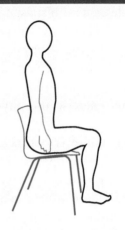
Standing • Feet flat on the floor. • Knees neither locked nor bent. • Abdominal muscles tight and buttocks tucked in. • Shoulders back and down slightly, even, and relaxed. • Head facing forward, not tilted to one side or the other. • Chin tucked and ears over the shoulders.	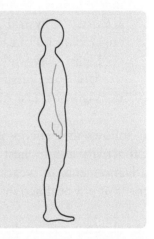
Sleeping • Posture is midline and symmetrical (i.e., the two sides are equal). • Sleeping in a supine position (on the back) is recommended. • If lying on one side, it can be helpful to place a pillow between the legs to keep the spine in good alignment. A pillow under the top arm can also be useful to support good alignment—often the top arm is pulled down by gravity, which can result in curving of the spine or rolling to prone position (sleeping on the front) in the night.	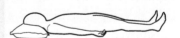

Exercise and physical activity

Exercise and physical activity are also constants in the life of the child and adolescent with spastic diplegia. The goal of exercise and physical activity for a person with spastic diplegia is the same as for their nondisabled peers. Having a physical disability does not confer any exemption from needing to exercise and stay physically active.

While exercise and physical activity are related, there are differences:

- **Exercise** is planned, structured, repetitive, and intentional movement to improve or maintain physical fitness.[202] Exercise is a subtype of physical activity. Examples of exercise include running, cycling, and attending a gym class.
- **Physical activity** is movement carried out by the skeletal muscles that requires energy expenditure; thus any movement is physical activity.[202] Physical activity varies from light to moderate to vigorous. Examples of each include:
  - Light: slow walking
  - Moderate: brisk walking, jogging, climbing stairs
  - Vigorous: fast running, fast cycling

It follows that energy expenditure is lowest while doing light physical activity and highest while doing vigorous physical activity. Recent advancements in wearable monitoring devices allow better measurement of physical activity levels in individuals with CP.[203,204]

Do children and adolescents with spastic diplegia take part in enough physical activity? No. Studies have shown that children with CP walk significantly less[205] and spend more time being sedentary[206] than typically developing children. A further study[204] found that children age 3 to 12 showed a decrease in amount and intensity of physical activity with increasing GMFCS level* and increasing age. Participants at GMFCS level I showed the steepest decrease with increasing age.

Does this reduced physical activity have health consequences? Yes. Reduced physical activity has been associated with higher energy cost

---

* Levels I and II compared with levels III to V combined.

of walking in adolescents with mild spastic CP[207] and elevated blood pressure in children and adolescents with mild or moderate spastic CP.[208]

Do studies show exercise and physical activity are beneficial for children and adolescents with CP? Again, yes. Studies have found benefits across a range of measures, including fitness, body composition, quality of life, and happiness.[209,210,211] A physical therapy research summit sponsored by the American Physical Therapy Association emphasized the need to promote and maintain physical fitness in children with CP to improve health, reduce secondary conditions, and enhance quality of life.[212]

Verschuren and colleagues published a set of exercise and physical activity recommendations for people with CP under the following headings:[213]

- Cardiorespiratory (aerobic) exercise
- Resistance (muscle strengthening) exercise
- Daily moderate to vigorous physical activity
- Avoiding sedentary behavior (i.e., not being physically inactive)

Table 3.5.2 summarizes their recommendations, which are similar to (and based on) the World Health Organization's guidelines for nondisabled people.[214] Though these recommendations are relatively recent, the concept that "exercise is medicine" is not new.[215] Note that these are lifetime recommendations; it may take at least 8 to 16 consecutive weeks of exercise to see the benefit.[213] Also note that there is no lower (or upper) age limit on the exercise and physical activity recommendations for people with CP.

There is no denying these recommendations are demanding. However, research has found that typically developing infants can take up to 9,000 steps in a given day and travel the equivalent of 29 football fields.[216] It is important to be aware of the recommendations and aim to meet them as much as possible. And remember, any activity is better than no activity.

Table 3.5.2 Exercise and physical activity recommendations for people with CP

TYPE OF EXERCISE/ PHYSICAL ACTIVITY	RECOMMENDATIONS FOR PEOPLE WITH CP	COMMENTS
Cardiorespiratory (aerobic) exercise Regular, purposeful exercise that involves major muscle groups and is continuous and rhythmic in nature	3 times per week > 60% of peak heart rate* Minimum of 20 minutes per session	This is the type of exercise that gets the heart pumping and the lungs working.
Resistance (muscle strengthening) exercise	2 to 4 times per week on nonconsecutive days	Muscle strengthening is especially important because muscle weakness is a feature of spastic CP.
Daily moderate to vigorous physical activity	60 minutes ≥ 5 days per week	This is the ordinary movement of everyday life. Physical activity counts as long as it is moderate to vigorous. It is less taxing than cardiorespiratory exercise but more vigorous than gentle movement. Walking, going up stairs, and household chores are all included in this category.
Avoiding sedentary behavior (not being physically inactive)	Sit for less than 2 hours a day or break up sitting for 2 minutes every 30 to 60 minutes	A person can be physically active but still sedentary; they are separately measured. For example, if the person meets the recommendation for moderate to vigorous physical activity but sits for long periods watching TV or playing computer games, then they are physically active but sedentary. Prolonged sitting in one position, particularly with bad posture, is not good for anyone.

* Peak heart rate can be approximated as 220 minus age. For example, at age 15, peak heart rate is 205 (220-15). Sixty percent of peak heart rate is approximately 120 beats/minute (205 x 0.6). *From Verschuren and colleagues.*[213]

The Peter Harrison Centre for Disability Sport at Loughborough University in the UK has published two excellent guides specifically for people of all ages with CP. The first, *Fit for Life*, is for people with CP who are new to exercise. The second, *Fit for Sport*, is for people who want to take their athletics to a more advanced level.[217,218] The first guide contains a very useful table, "What type of exercise can I do?" listing advantages and disadvantages with adaptations and advice for each type of exercise. One of the advantages noted is that almost all can be done in the community with peers. Many children and adolescents with CP appreciate doing exercise in regular settings rather than as part of therapy. Both guides are included in **Useful web resources.**

Another resource is World Abilitysport, an international organization for the development of para sports—competitive sports specifically designed or adapted for individuals with physical, sensory, or intellectual disability.[219] Figure 3.5.1 shows World Abilitysport's list of sports and para sports for individuals with CP across GMFCS levels.

	GMFCS I 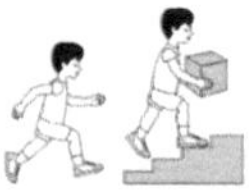	GMFCS II 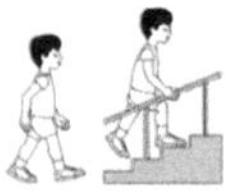
Athletics	Ambulant Athletics – Track and Field	Ambulant Athletics - Track and Field
Swimming	Unaided swimming	Unaided swimming
Football	CP 7-a-side Football	CP 7-a-side Football
Racquet Sports	Standing Badminton Standing Table-Tennis Standing Cricket	Standing Badminton Standing Table-Tennis Standing Cricket Wheelchair Tennis
Individual Sports	Taekwondo Para-Cycling (2/3 wheeler) Para Triathlon Equestrian CP Bowls Standing Archery standing Golf Para Shooting Powerlifting Seated Fencing	Taekwondo Para-Cycling (2/3 wheeler) Para Triathlon Equestrian CP Bowls Standing Archery standing Golf Para Shooting Powerlifting Seated Fencing
Team Sports	Sitting Volleyball Beach ParaVolley Ambulant CP rugby Ambulant Netball	Sitting Volleyball Beach ParaVolley Ambulant CP rugby Ambulant Netball
Winter Sports	Standing Alpine Skiing Standing Nordic Skiing Snowboarding Para Ice Hockey	Standing Alpine Skiing Standing Nordic Skiing Snowboarding Para Ice Hockey
Water Sports	Rowing Sailing Canoeing	Rowing Sailing Canoeing

Figure 3.5.1 Sports and para sports for individuals with CP across the GMFCS levels. Reproduced with kind permission from World Abilitysport. GMFCS illustrations Version 2 © Bill Reid, Kate Willoughby, Adrienne Harvey, and Kerr Graham, The Royal Children's Hospital Melbourne.

GMFCS III	GMFCS IV	GMFCS V
RaceRunning Seated Athletics - Track and Field	RaceRunning Seated Athletics - Track and Field	RaceRunning Seated Athletics – Track and Field
Unaided swimming		
Frame Football	Frame Football Powerchair Football	Powerchair Football
Wheelchair Badminton Wheelchair Tennis Seated Table Tennis Wheelchair Cricket	Wheelchair Badminton Wheelchair Tennis Seated Table Tennis Table Cricket	Table Cricket
Para-Cycling (2/3 wheeler) Seated Fencing Para Triathlon Boccia Equestrian CP Bowls Seated Archery seated Wheelchair Slalom Para Shooting Powerlifting	Para-Cycling (2/3 wheeler) Seated Fencing Boccia CP Bowls Seated Archery seated Para Shooting Powerlifting Trap Driving Wheelchair Slalom	Wheelchair Slalom Boccia Para Shooting Trap Driving
Sitting Volleyball Wheelchair Basketball Wheelchair Rugby	Sitting Volleyball Wheelchair Basketball Wheelchair Rugby	
Sitting Alpine Skiing Standing/Sitting Nordic Skiing Wheelchair Curling Para Ice Hockey	Sitting Nordic Skiing Wheelchair Curling	
Rowing Sailing Canoeing	Sailing Canoeing	Assisted Sailing

Further tips on exercise and physical activity are included in Appendix 5 (online). An appointment with a physical therapist, occupational therapist, or a recreational therapist is useful if further guidance is needed on how to create an exercise program that suits the needs and abilities of the individual.

If you think being good at exercise and sports is impossible for the person with spastic diplegia, think again. Rixt van der Horst is a Dutch Paralympian with spastic diplegia who competes in dressage.* Rowan Crothers, an Australian Paralympic swimmer, and Brianna Salinaro, a US Paralympian who competes in tae kwon do, also have spastic diplegia. These athletes are proof that spastic diplegia is not a barrier to achieving great levels of fitness and skill.

Daniel Dias, retired Brazilian Paralympic swimmer who won multiple medals, credited fellow retired Paralympian Clodoaldo Silva, who has CP, for getting him into the sport. "I only began because I saw Clodoaldo swimming on television. I didn't know people like me could swim, could do any sport at all."[220]

Paralympians include people with a range of types and levels of disabilities. Many Paralympic athletes are able to swim, cycle, and run faster than their average nondisabled peers. For example, at the Brazil 2016 games, four Paralympic runners beat the time of the Olympic gold medalist in the men's 1,500 meters.[221] US Paralympians now train with Olympic athletes at US Olympic and Paralympic Committee training centers under the supervision of the same coaches. The guiding principle of the Paralympic movement is to keep competition as fair as possible, and classification is the cornerstone. Classification is sport specific because an individual's impairment may affect their ability to perform in different sports to a different extent. For example, in swimming:

> *There are ten different sport classes for athletes with physical impairment, numbered 1-10. Athletes with different impairments compete against each other, because sport classes are allocated based on the impact the impairment has on swimming, rather than on the impairment itself. To evaluate the impact of impairments on swimming, classifiers assess all functional body*

---

* In dressage, a horse and rider perform a series of predetermined movements.

structures using a point system and ask the athlete to complete a water assessment.[222]

There are currently 28 Paralympic sports sanctioned by the International Paralympic Committee: 22 summer and 6 winter sports.[222]

Summer sports:

- Para archery
- Para athletics
- Para badminton
- Blind football (for athletes with a vision impairment)
- Boccia
- Para canoe
- Para cycling
- Para equestrian
- Goalball (for athletes with a vision impairment)
- Para judo (for athletes with a vision impairment)
- Para powerlifting
- Para rowing
- Shooting para sport
- Sitting volleyball
- Para swimming
- Para table tennis
- Para tae kwon do
- Para triathlon
- Wheelchair basketball
- Wheelchair fencing
- Wheelchair rugby
- Wheelchair tennis

Winter sports:

- Para alpine skiing
- Para biathlon
- Para cross-country skiing
- Para ice hockey
- Para snowboard
- Wheelchair curling

Links to various organizations are included in **Useful web resources.**

Good exercise and physical activity habits start early in life. Children are much more likely to have good habits if their parents do, and they are much more likely to have good habits as adults if they had good habits as children. The habits we parents keep, and the habits we instill in our children, have lifelong effects on our children's adult health. The good news is that it is never too late to start.

Exercise and physical activity are part of the lifelong home program for people with spastic diplegia. However, it is worth acknowledging that many people (including those without a disability) do not meet the recommendations for exercise and physical activity. People with spastic diplegia may be at greater risk of an inactive lifestyle for many reasons, including overprotective parents (we may fear our child might get hurt) and difficulties with movement.

In Chapter 2, we addressed the unfavorable strength-to-mass ratio that develops as the child grows. It is therefore very important that the child with spastic diplegia enter the adolescent growth spurt with strong muscles and no excess weight. The home program can help with both.

Assistive technology

Determine that the thing can and shall be done,
and then we shall find the way.
Abraham Lincoln

Assistive technology refers to products and services designed to enhance the functional capabilities and independence of individuals with disabilities to allow them to participate.[223] This section addresses the following assistive technology commonly used by individuals with spastic diplegia:

- Orthoses
- Mobility aids
- Adaptive recreational equipment

Assistive technology should be selected based on assessments performed by a multidisciplinary team, including professionals (e.g., physician, physical and occupational therapists, orthotist) in conjunction with the individual and their family. An individual's unique health needs and the family's care and function goals help guide what assistive technology is best suited for the individual. Regular reevaluation is important, the frequency of which depends on the individual and the product.[*]

Orthoses

An orthosis is a device designed to hold specific body parts in position in order to modify their structure and/or function. The term "orthosis" comes from the Greek word "ortho," which means "to straighten or align." Orthotics is the branch of medicine concerned with the design, manufacture, and management of orthoses. The orthotist is the professional in this specialty. The word "orthotic" is sometimes used to mean the device; "orthosis" is the more correct term, but given how alike the two terms are, their interchangeability is understandable. The terms "brace" and "splint" are also sometimes used.

Orthoses work best when a child has no contractures or bone torsions, though many children with spastic diplegia may have both; then, orthoses can at least be partially effective as long as they are not too cumbersome or limiting.

Different orthoses have different functions. The goals of treatment with orthoses may include the following:[224]

- Maintain or improve ROM at a joint through a prolonged stretch
- Provide stability or support to a joint
- Improve function of a limb
- Improve balance
- Improve gait
- Provide protection
- Accommodate or minimize a joint alignment problem
- Prepare for surgery
- Facilitate positioning after surgery

---

[*] In the US, some assistive technology is referred to as "durable medical equipment" (DME) for medical insurance purposes.

There is often a trade-off or competing goals with orthoses. For example, the best orthosis for walking may not be the best for getting up and down from the floor, and using an orthosis to protect or correctly align a body part may decrease muscle strength. For this reason, if the orthosis includes the ankle joint, the child or adolescent should also spend some time out of the orthosis since it is important to maintain strength in the muscles that don't have to work when it is worn; in this case the muscles of the dorsiflexors (shin) and plantar flexors (calf). Additionally, different orthoses may be prescribed over the years as the child or adolescent grows and their body structure and function changes. As a result, collaborative goal-setting is important, and choosing an orthosis can involve different specialists on the multidisciplinary team.[225]

Orthoses can be custom-made (molded to a specific individual's body) or prefabricated (fit based on size and already made). Once a device has been prescribed, the individual will be evaluated and a device may be fitted the same day if it is prefabricated and readily available. A device such as a custom-made ankle-foot orthosis (AFO) requires a mold to be taken and a return visit after a few weeks for a fitting. Adjustments are made to confirm that it is comfortable and functions well. Adhering to the prescribed wear time is critical to ensure that the individual receives the full benefit of the device. After the initial fitting, further adjustments may be needed if the individual is experiencing:

- Discomfort
- Redness
- Skin breakdown
- A growth spurt
- A change in functionality
- A change in ROM

Additionally, children will likely outgrow their devices before they wear them out and may require new devices every year or so until they stop growing.

Lower extremity orthoses are used for the feet, ankles, knees, and hips. They are intended to maintain or improve ROM at the joint, provide support and stability, improve function and gait, and more. The following lower extremity orthoses may be used in spastic diplegia and are described in Table 3.6.1.

- Foot orthosis (FO)
- Supramalleolar orthosis (SMO)
- Ankle-foot orthosis (AFO)
- Knee immobilizer (KI)
- Knee orthosis (KO)

Having well-fitting shoes is a must when wearing orthoses intended for standing or walking. If the shoes do not fit well or are worn out, the orthoses may not function correctly and may not be comfortable. In most cases, a slightly larger shoe is needed. Certain stores, including some online, allow purchase of two different-size shoes. Athletic shoes that can be zipped, laced, or fastened snugly can be a good option. Some manufacturers of athletic shoes now offer models that are specifically designed to be easy to get on and off with orthoses, such as some BILLY shoes or the Nike FlyEase.

Table 3.6.1 Common lower extremity orthoses for individuals with spastic diplegia

ORTHOSIS TYPE	SUBTYPE	DESCRIPTION
Foot orthosis (FO)	Functional or accommodative	FOs are semi-rigid custom-molded shoe inserts. They replace regular shoe insoles and can be left in the shoes. Accommodative FOs cushion or protect a rigid foot or a foot that lacks sensation; functional FOs provide support and help maintain proper alignment.
	University of California-Berkeley Lab (UCBL)	A UCBL orthosis, similar to the functional FO, supports, distributes pressure, and helps maintain proper foot alignment. However, the UCBL is taller and is made of more rigid plastic to provide greater support. UCBLs usually replace regular insoles and can be left in the shoes.
Supramalleolar orthosis (SMO)		A supramalleolar orthosis ("supra" means "above" and "malleolar" refers to the bony prominences of the ankle), extends just above the ankle. As with FOs and UCBLs, the SMO controls the foot. However, as the SMO also captures the ankle joint, it exerts greater control and provides additional support and stability.

Cont'd.

ORTHOSIS TYPE	SUBTYPE	DESCRIPTION
Ankle-foot orthosis (AFO) An AFO extends above the ankle joint and stops before the knee. It protects the foot, manages foot malalignments, prevents the toes from dragging during gait, provides varying levels of support and stability to the ankle and/or knee during standing and walking, and prevents the progression of ankle muscle contractures.	Articulated AFO 	An articulated AFO has a hinge at the ankle joint to allow free dorsiflexion (moving the foot up). It often has a plastic posterior "stop" that blocks plantar flexion, preventing the user from moving the foot down or dragging their toes. Free dorsiflexion allows the user to easily rise to standing from the floor, transition from one position to another, and climb stairs. Articulated AFOs are also worn by adolescents and adults who would benefit from the added ROM while still preventing their toes from dragging.
	Posterior leaf spring (PLS) AFO 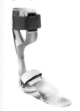	The PLS AFO has a calf cuff that tapers to a thinner strut behind the ankle. It prevents toes from dragging and restricts dorsiflexion, the amount of which depends on the width and stiffness of the posterior strut. Because the sides are trimmed back, it may not be the best choice for someone who requires significant ankle and/or knee support or who has severe joint contractures.
	Solid AFO (SAFO) 	A SAFO is the most supportive type of AFO. It is typically made of a rigid, durable plastic and provides maximum stability for the ankle and knee. This AFO does not allow ankle movement, which can make some functional movements difficult to perform while wearing it (e.g., going up and down stairs). It is most often recommended for individuals with severe tone, muscle contractures, or bony malalignments.
	Ground reaction AFO (GRAFO) or floor reaction AFO (FRAFO) 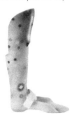	The GRAFO is a solid AFO with an additional anterior shell. The solid ankle design provides maximum control at the ankle, and the anterior shell forces the knee to extend, helping to limit crouch gait. The GRAFO can sometimes be difficult to put on and take off because the foot has to be inserted from the rear. It is ineffective for use with knee or hip flexion contractures because the knee cannot completely straighten.

Cont'd.

ORTHOSIS TYPE	SUBTYPE	DESCRIPTION
Ankle-foot orthosis (AFO) *Cont'd*	Carbon fiber AFO	A carbon fiber AFO can be prefabricated or custom-made. It may have a posterior strut similar to a PLS AFO (top image) or an anterior shell similar to a GRAFO (bottom image). Prefabricated designs will prevent toes from dragging and provide light support while the carbon material provides energy return to the user. Custom-made carbon fiber AFOs may provide additional support for high-level activities.
	Nighttime AFO or stretching splint	A prefabricated nighttime AFO typically has a plastic shell, soft inner liner, and adjustable straps. It is worn just at night and is designed to help stretch the calf muscles, maintain ankle ROM, and prevent the progression of ankle muscle contractures.
Knee immobilizer (KI)		A KI consists of a soft knee wrap, rigid aluminum struts, and straps to adjust the fit. As the name suggests, the KI prevents the knee from moving. It is used to stretch the knee flexors (hamstrings) or to maintain ROM after surgery.

Cont'd.

ORTHOSIS TYPE	SUBTYPE	DESCRIPTION
Knee orthosis (KO)	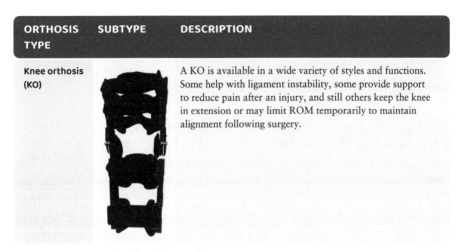	A KO is available in a wide variety of styles and functions. Some help with ligament instability, some provide support to reduce pain after an injury, and still others keep the knee in extension or may limit ROM temporarily to maintain alignment following surgery.

Adapted from Ward and colleagues.[224]

Research supports the use of AFOs for improved stride length[*] and ankle movement.[14]

To get a child to consistently wear an orthosis, it must be comfortable; it must not cause any rubbing or blisters, for example. You should not hesitate to speak up if you notice any problems, even minor ones.

Orthoses must also be acceptable in appearance to the wearer. It helps if they can choose from a variety of colors and designs. An orthosis would not (and should not) be prescribed unless it's necessary, so although the child may not love wearing it, they should wear it as prescribed. A child may not like being restrained in a car seat, but we don't give them the option of not wearing a seat belt. We really have to adopt the same approach when it comes to orthoses (within reason); it's what's best for the child in the long term. We have to be both good cop and bad cop at once.

Thankfully, Tommy never objected to wearing orthoses. Over the years he was prescribed different types, including FOs, UCBLs, SMOs, and articulated and solid AFOs. Being able to choose from different colors and designs certainly helped—though I didn't love the American flag

---

[*] Stride length is the distance covered from one heel strike to the next heel strike of the same foot. In other words, it is equal to two steps, one for each foot.

design he chose for his AFOs after orthopedic surgery in the US—I wanted to be diplomatic when we returned to our home health care services after having chosen an alternate treatment route. The two American flags on Tommy's calves didn't exactly help!

The only real problem we encountered with orthoses was when Tommy left Ireland for college in the US. We tried to make sure he was well prepared, which included getting new orthoses (in this case, SMOs). The orthoses arrived just a few days before he was due to leave. He'd never had problems with new orthoses before, but this time he developed large blisters on the soles of both feet. A nurse friend dressed his feet each night to allow him to walk easily by day. When he left for college, I was honestly more worried about the blisters on his feet than anything else. We dropped him off at his dorm, and the following day we checked out the college medical center. The staff assured him (well, mostly me) that they would be available any time he needed them. Thankfully, both Tommy and his new orthoses settled in just fine.

AFOs were recommended early on in Tommy's treatment. At the time, I had no idea what they were. The term "AFO" was new to me, and it's not exactly self-explanatory. To me, they sounded like UFOs!

Mobility aids

Although individuals with spastic diplegia GMFCS levels I to III are able to walk, those at GMFCS levels II and III may need a cane and crutches for safety and balance, and wheeled mobility for traveling long distance so as not to fatigue easily. As addressed in section 3.4, navigating high school and college campuses can involve a lot of walking, and there is a balance to be struck between independent walking and using walking/mobility aids (such as a cane, walker, or a wheelchair). Mobility aids may reduce fatigue and/or pain with walking to allow the child or adolescent to participate more in everyday life safely and with more energy available that is not spent on walking alone.

Mobility aids discussed here include:

a) Canes and crutches
b) Walkers
c) Gait trainers
d) Scooters
e) Wheelchairs

a) Canes and crutches

A cane (walking stick) is an aid that typically consists of a handle at the top, a shaft, and a tip that makes contact with the ground. Canes can be single-pronged (straight cane), three-pronged (tripod cane), or four-pronged (quad cane). Tripod and quad canes provide more balance than a straight cane, and children typically use them rather than straight canes. See Figure 3.6.1.

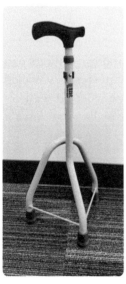 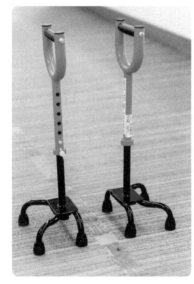

Figure 3.6.1 Pediatric tripod cane (left) and quad canes (right).

A crutch is similar to a cane but provides more support. The individual leans on the crutch and uses their arms and hands to support a significant portion of their body weight. Crutches can be used singly or in pairs. Armpit (axillary) crutches have padded rests that sit under the armpits, while forearm crutches (also known as lofstrand crutches), have arm cuffs that cover the forearms. See Figures 3.6.2 and 3.6.3.

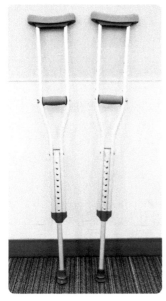 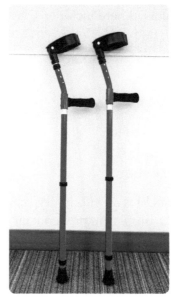

Figure 3.6.2 Armpit crutches.   **Figure 3.6.3** Forearm crutches.

b) Walkers

Walkers typically consist of a wheeled frame with handles. Walkers can be forward-wheeled (walker in front of the user) or posterior-wheeled (walker behind the user). (See Figure 3.6.4.) Posterior-wheeled walkers are more commonly used with children. A posterior walker can have a fold down seat that allows a child who easily tires to take a rest.[224]

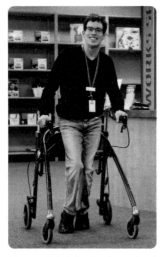

Figure 3.6.4 Posterior-wheeled walker.

c) Gait trainers

A gait trainer is similar to a walker but offers increased postural support, weight-bearing capabilities, and mobility assistance while walking. Gait trainers typically consist of a wheeled frame with weight-bearing support straps and upper extremity supports such as a tray, handle, or handrail. See Figure 3.6.5.

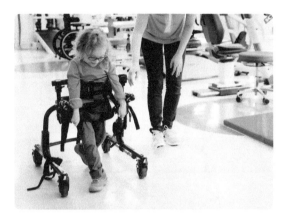

Figure 3.6.5 Gait trainer.

d) Scooters

Scooters are motorized mobility devices that typically have a seat and handlebars for steering, and electric-powered wheels that allow the user to navigate indoors or outdoors. See Figure 3.6.6.

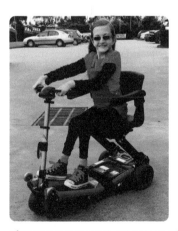

Figure 3.6.6 Motorized scooter for mobility. Reproduced with kind permission from Mounties Care.

e) Wheelchairs

Table 3.6.2 summarizes different wheelchair types.

Table 3.6.2 Wheelchairs

TYPE	DESCRIPTION
Manual wheelchair	A manual wheelchair is self-propelled by the individual or pushed by a caregiver. Thus, independent mobility with a manual wheelchair requires a degree of upper extremity motor control and strength.
Power-assist wheelchair	A power-assist wheelchair (also known as a power-assisted wheelchair or a power add-on) is designed to enhance the manual propulsion of a standard wheelchair. It provides an extra power boost to the user's manual efforts, making it easier to propel the wheelchair over various terrains or inclines. The power-assist feature is typically incorporated into the wheels either as an integrated system or as an attachable device.
Power wheelchair	A power wheelchair (also known as an electric wheelchair or motorized wheelchair) is powered by an electric motor that is controlled by an electronic control system (joystick, buttons, or other devices). It is worth noting that a power wheelchair is a heavy machine and cannot be lifted like a manual wheelchair.

Adaptive recreational equipment

A variety of adaptive recreational equipment is available to make participation in various recreational or leisure pursuits possible or just easier. An appointment with a recreational therapist, physical therapist, or occupational therapist is useful if people need guidance. Examples of such equipment include:

a) Adaptive cycles
b) Adaptive workout equipment
c) Hiking aids
d) Other outdoor and adventure sports equipment

a) Adaptive cycles

Adaptive cycles come in many configurations, but for the individual with spastic diplegia, a tricycle provides more stability because it compensates for balance challenges. See Figures 3.6.7 and 3.6.8.

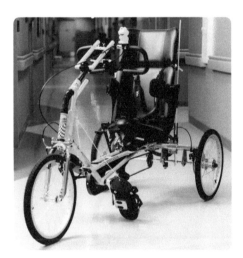

Figure 3.6.7 A foot-powered adaptive tricycle.

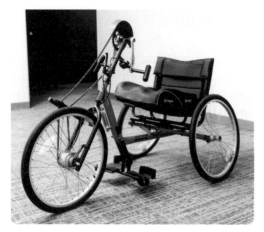

Figure 3.6.8 A hand-powered adaptive tricycle.

The following accessories may be helpful:

- Footplates (sometimes called shoe holders) with straps to keep the feet on the pedals (shown in Figures 3.6.7 and 3.6.8)
- Leg calipers (braces attached to the pedals) to keep the leg in the correct position
- Pulleys (strings attached to the front of the pedals) to adjust the rider's dorsiflexion (shown in Figure 3.6.7)
- Electric assist to compensate for endurance or rides of long duration (dependent on responsibility of rider)
- Caregiver steering control to help in circumstances when braking or turning is more difficult (on sidewalks, near traffic, down declines)

b) Adaptive workout equipment

Weight-lifting exercises may be done safely with adaptive equipment such as a wrist cuff grip to hold a free weight. They can also be done with a regular wrist weight that goes around the wrist or by using resistance bands. See Figure 3.6.9.

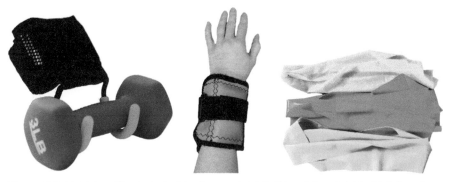

Figure 3.6.9 Wrist cuff grip to hold a free weight (left), wrist weight (middle), and resistance bands (right).

c) Hiking aids

Many individuals with spastic diplegia can use hiking poles to correct for their balance challenges on uneven terrain. A track chair can also allow participation. A track chair is an all-terrain wheelchair that can safely navigate outdoor spaces when mobility problems make it otherwise unsafe to enjoy the activity. Some large parks and recreational facilities have these chairs available to borrow while at the park or beach, for example.

d) Other outdoor and adventure sports equipment

Adaptive equipment is available for many other outdoor and adventure sports, including:

- Snow skiing (e.g., outriggers)
- Waterskiing (e.g., arm sling handles, shoulder wraps, sit skis)
- Golf (e.g., adaptive club grips and golf carts)
- Kayaking (e.g., angled oars, outriggers, trolling motors)
- Surfing (e.g., specialized systems)
- Horseback riding (e.g., high back saddles for balance)

See Figure 3.6.10.

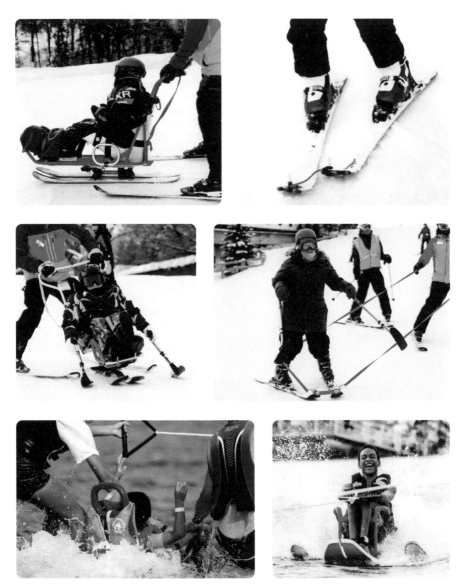

Figure 3.6.10 Adaptive snow skiing and waterskiing with various levels of assistance and support.

If there is upper limb involvement, various adaptive equipment is available to help improve function. More information on adaptive recreational equipment is included in Appendix 2 (online).

Tone reduction

The good physician treats the disease; the great
physician treats the patient who has the disease.

Sir William Osler

Abnormal muscle tone is addressed in section 2.6. To recap: Muscle tone is the resting tension in a person's muscles. A range of "normal" muscle tone exists. Tone is considered "abnormal" when it falls outside the range of normal or typical. Abnormal muscle tone occurs in all types of CP. Spasticity is the main type of high tone in spastic diplegia, but dystonia may also occur. Data from the Australian CP register shows that 12 percent of individuals with spastic diplegia (all GMFCS levels) have co-occurring dyskinesia, 2 percent have co-occurring ataxia, and 1 percent have co-occurring hypotonia,[*][42] and it is believed that the true prevalence of co-occurring motor types is higher.[4]

Spasticity is defined as an abnormal increase in muscle tone or stiffness of muscle that can interfere with movement and speech, and be associated with discomfort or pain.[22] Another definition highlights the

---

* For those who acquired CP in the pre- or perinatal period only.

velocity-dependent nature of the condition.[104] Dystonia, a type of dyskinesia, is characterized by involuntary (unintended) muscle contractions that cause slow repetitive movements or abnormal postures that can sometimes be painful.[39]

Tone reduction is a high priority in the early years. However, tone reduction is only one part of the integrated treatment of spastic diplegia by the multidisciplinary team. It is usually performed in conjunction with other treatments such as PT, OT, serial casting, and orthoses. When tone reduction is included with other treatments, the effects of each treatment may be amplified—the combination of treatments may be more effective than any one treatment on its own.

Reducing spasticity helps reduce the harmful effects of high tone on skeletal growth. It also helps reduce stiffness and increases the overall ROM of joints. Increasing the ROM a person can move through facilitates strengthening, working on motor control, balance, and other functional goals. It can also improve a person's tolerance for wearing orthoses.

Table 3.7.1 lists tone reduction treatments commonly used in individuals with spastic diplegia.

The AACPDM (American Academy for Cerebral Palsy and Developmental Medicine) has published a care pathway, "Cerebral Palsy and Dystonia"; a link to it is included in **Useful web resources.**

Table 3.7.1 Tone reduction treatments

TREATMENT	TONE TYPE	AREA OF EFFECT **Generalized** = treatment affects a large region of the body. **Focal** = treatment has an effect on a local area (e.g., a single muscle)	DURATION OF EFFECT
Oral medications (medications taken by mouth)	Spasticity and dystonia	Generalized	Temporary
Botulinum neurotoxin A (BoNT-A) injection	Spasticity	Focal: injected into muscles	Temporary
Phenol injection	Spasticity	Focal: injected around nerves that control spastic muscles	Temporary
Intrathecal baclofen (ITB)	Spasticity and dystonia	Generalized	Temporary
Selective dorsal rhizotomy (SDR)	Spasticity	Generalized	Permanent

Many medical centers have special team evaluations for spasticity treatment planning because of its complexity and significance in CP. At Gillette Children's, for example, a spasticity evaluation involves a multidisciplinary team within a specialty spasticity evaluation clinic. The team includes professionals from physical medicine and rehabilitation (PM&R), orthopedics, and neurosurgery. The specialists see the child together, not individually, and come to a consensus on the best spasticity treatment for the child. The evaluation includes a gait analysis and functional PT assessment completed as part of the (typically) two-day evaluation. Spasticity clinics at other facilities may include additional team members from other specialties, including neurology and developmental pediatrics.

Different medical centers have different protocols for how they perform each tone-reducing treatment. For example, the selection criteria (for those for whom the treatment is suitable) and protocols (how the treatment is actually carried out) for SDR vary[226,227,228] which is why SDR is not a uniform procedure.* (Indeed, this point applies to all treatments in CP.)

As with all treatments for spastic diplegia, clear goals for tone reduction and assessment of outcome are required. Because the child has to adjust to their new, relaxed muscles, they may initially experience perceived weakness or temporary loss of function. Though the use of tone reduction treatment peaks in early childhood, it can continue into adolescence and adulthood.

We now look at the different tone reduction treatments in more detail.

Oral medications

Oral medications (those taken by mouth) are used to achieve generalized tone reduction. There are several oral medications physicians may prescribe to reduce high tone,[229] including:

- Baclofen
- Diazepam
- Dantrolene
- Tizanidine

These medications may have different brand names in different countries. They act on different sites in the body, with different effects on the muscles, brain, or spinal cord.[229]

The challenge of treatment with oral medications is balancing their side effects with their efficacy; benefits are greater for some people than for others. The medications are sometimes used in combination or in conjunction with focal spasticity reduction measures such as BoNT-A. They can also be used episodically to reduce muscle spasms after orthopedic surgery, for instance.

---

* Grunt and colleagues recommend that international meetings of experts should develop more uniform consensus guidelines.[226]

Research supports use of diazepam (green light) and dantrolene and tizanidine (yellow light) for reduced spasticity. Research supports use of oral baclofen for reduced spasticity and/or dystonia (yellow light).[14]

Botulinum neurotoxin A injection

Botulinum neurotoxin A (BoNT-A), as a medication, is injected directly into the muscle and acts by blocking the release of a chemical called acetylcholine at the neuromuscular junction (where the nerve meets the muscle). Botulinum neurotoxin* is produced by the bacteria that causes botulism, a lethal form of food poisoning. However, as a medication, the purified toxin is delivered at a much smaller dose. There are seven different types of botulinum neurotoxin, from A to G. Type A is the main form used to reduce spasticity.[230]

The effects of BoNT-A become apparent approximately three to seven days after injection and last for approximately three to six months.[231] The age at which treatment with BoNT-A begins varies among medical centers, with peak use between two and six years of age.[231] Protocols for use of BoNT-A (e.g., dosage and frequency of injection) also are different.[232] The effects of BoNT-A diminish with time. The original nerves regain their ability to release acetylcholine, but conflicting evidence exists on its long-term effect on the muscle itself.[230,231]

Several muscles may be treated in one session, although there is a limit to the total body dose of BoNT-A that can be safely given at one time.[230] Depending on the age of the individual and the number of muscles being injected, anesthesia may be required. Typically, no overnight hospital stay is necessary.

As with any injection, there may be some pain associated with the needle puncturing the skin and the delivery of the medicine. Different centers use different methods to manage pain; these may include distraction techniques (e.g., watching a video), topical or oral medication, nitrous oxide (laughing gas), or general anesthesia. Some children may experience stress and anxiety from repeated episodes of injection. One

---

* A poison that acts on the nervous system.

limiting factor of this treatment is the possibility of diminishing effect with repeat injections, or it may stop being effective entirely.[230]

The simultaneous use of BoNT-A and strength training has been found to be successful at reducing spasticity, improving strength, and achieving functional goals over and above treatment with BoNT-A alone.[233] This is an example of combined treatments working better together.

While there is strong evidence supporting BoNT-A treatment,[14,234,235] concerns are being raised. BoNT-A is regarded as a temporary treatment for reducing spasticity, but important questions have been asked about its long-term effects, including muscle weakness, muscle atrophy (wastage), changes in the muscle structure, and atrophy of the underlying bone.[3,231,236–242] Some studies suggest there may be permanent changes. For example, Multani and colleagues reported that human volunteers and experimental animals show muscle atrophy for at least 12 months after BoNT-A treatment.[231] They added that "muscle atrophy was accompanied by loss of contractile elements in muscle and replacement with fat and connective tissue," and that it was not currently known if these changes are reversible. They concluded that there is a need to use BoNT-A "more thoughtfully, less frequently and with greatly enhanced monitoring of the effects on injected muscle for both short-term and long-term benefits and harms."[231]

Tommy had BoNT-A injections on two or three occasions as a young child. We didn't notice any major changes following these injections. Unfortunately, however, it was not clear to me back then how to best use the time after injection. I regret that by the time I learned of SDR when he was nine years old, he had missed out on what would have been a treatment of choice. At an earlier age, he would have met the "ideal" candidate criteria for SDR, but by age nine he already needed orthopedic surgery to address his muscle and bone problems.

Phenol injection

Phenol is another medication delivered by injection. It was used as a treatment for spasticity for many decades before the advent of BoNT-A.

Phenol is injected directly around the motor nerve,[*] causing a breakdown of the insulation around the nerve, which prevents it from sending messages to the muscle. (Note that phenol is injected around the nerve, whereas BoNT-A is injected into the muscle.) Treatment with phenol is normally done under general anesthesia to minimize both discomfort for the patient and movement during the injection process. Usually, two to four muscle groups are injected in a single session.

Side effects of phenol may include paresthesia (a pins-and-needles or burning sensation if sensory nerves are affected instead of just the motor nerves) and weakness. The paresthesia may last a few weeks and is treated with gabapentin. The weakness usually resolves within two to four weeks. Again, no overnight hospital stay is typically necessary.

The effects of phenol generally last 3 to 12 months. Repeated injections can lead to a cumulative effect, meaning longer than one year,[230] but this is not common.

The use of phenol differs around the world. It has become less popular for a number of reasons, including the advent of BoNT-A,[230] Sometimes it is used in conjunction with BoNT-A because it allows more muscles to be treated without exceeding the dosage recommendations for either medication.[201] Some centers may use other alcohols in addition to phenol.

There is only one study of phenol use in CP,[14] which points to the lack of research evidence, but clinical expertise supports its use.

Intrathecal baclofen

Intrathecal baclofen (ITB) is another method for delivering the medication baclofen as a tone-reducing treatment for both spasticity and dystonia. It is generally better at reducing tone in the lower extremities than the upper extremities.[243]

---

[*] A nerve that sends signals away from the brain and spinal cord to a muscle; contrast with a sensory nerve, which sends signals (about temperature, pain, touch, etc.) from all parts of the body to the spinal cord and brain.

The following is an explanation of each term:

- **Intrathecal:** "Intra" means "within," and the "theca" is the sheath enclosing the spinal cord. The intrathecal area is the fluid-filled space surrounding the spinal cord; cerebrospinal fluid flows through this area, bathing and protecting the spinal cord.
- **Baclofen:** The name of the medication.

With ITB, a pump stores and delivers baclofen directly to the cerebrospinal fluid in the intrathecal space. Implanting an ITB pump is a surgical procedure. The pump is filled with baclofen and inserted under the skin and its soft tissue layer, typically in the abdomen. A catheter (a narrow, flexible tube) is connected to the pump and routed under the skin and its soft tissue layer to the patient's back. Surgeons make an incision to thread and position the tip of the catheter in the intrathecal space, where it delivers the baclofen directly to the cerebrospinal fluid. The pump is programmed to slowly release baclofen either in a consistent dose or in bursts of medication over a 24-hour period, depending on which method best helps the individual's high tone.[244] See Figure 3.7.1.

Delivering baclofen directly into the cerebrospinal fluid is much more effective and requires a much lower dose (about one-thousandth of the oral dose). It can help avoid or minimize side effects that individuals may experience when taking oral baclofen such as dizziness and drowsiness.

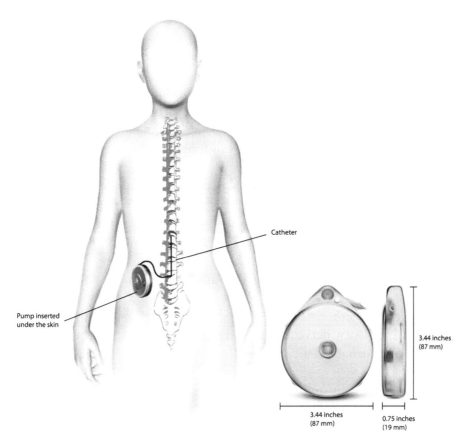

Figure 3.7.1 Intrathecal baclofen.

Implanting an ITB pump usually requires a hospital stay, typically five to seven days. It is important for the patient to lie flat for up to three days afterwards to allow the surgical site to heal and avoid spinal fluid from leaking. The patient wears an abdominal binder for six to eight weeks afterward to support the pump and prevent swelling.[244] The pump has to be refilled with baclofen about every three to four months, on average, in an outpatient clinic. The pump runs on a battery that has a limited life, requiring the pump to be surgically removed and replaced after about seven years. This can usually be done with an overnight hospital stay.

Research supports the use of ITB for reduced spasticity and/or dystonia and other outcomes (green and yellow lights).[14]

Selective dorsal rhizotomy

Selective dorsal rhizotomy (SDR) is a neurosurgical procedure that reduces spasticity by selectively cutting abnormal sensory nerve root-lets* in the spinal cord. SDR reduces spasticity only, not other types of high tone. It is an irreversible tone-reducing treatment. The following is an explanation of each word in the full term:

- **Selective:** Only certain abnormal nerve rootlets are cut.
- **Dorsal:** "Dorsal" refers to the sensory nerve rootlets. (They are termed "dorsal" because they are located toward the back of the body. The motor nerve rootlets are termed "ventral" because they are toward the front.)
- **Rhizotomy:** "Rhizo" means "root," and "otomy" means "to cut into."

Putting it all together, "selective dorsal rhizotomy" means that certain abnormal, sensory nerve rootlets are cut to diminish the overactive reflex loop causing spasticity.

There are generally two SDR techniques, the cauda and the conus, named after the level of the spinal cord at which each procedure is performed. The choice of technique is surgeon-specific but also depends on the patient. The cauda technique is the most common worldwide.[226] Similar short-term gait and functional outcomes have been reported with each technique.[245]

SDR involves removing the back of the vertebrae (the lamina) to access the spinal cord. This is called a "laminectomy." During the operation, the sensory (dorsal) nerve roots are dissected into their individual root-lets. The rootlets are then individually electrically stimulated to deter-mine whether they trigger a normal or abnormal (spastic) response. If a rootlet triggers an abnormal response, it is cut. If not, it is left alone. The percentage of rootlets cut varies among medical centers.[226] At Gillette Children's, the percentage of rootlets cut during SDR is lower than what is typically reported in the literature. If too high a percentage of rootlets are cut, there is greater risk of inducing weakness.

---

* Think of a stick of string cheese, or a telephone cable with many smaller wires together in it. The nerve root is the whole cheese stick, or the whole telephone cable, and the smaller cheese strings or wires within the cable are the rootlets.

As with many treatments, SDR is not suitable for every child. The selection criteria for SDR differs among medical centers.[226] As an example, characteristics of the "ideal" candidate for SDR at Gillette Children's include.*[246]

- Age four to seven years
- GMFCS level I–III
- Primarily spasticity (as opposed to dystonia) that interferes with function and involves multiple muscles and joints in the lower limbs
- Preterm birth history or injury in the late second or early third trimester of pregnancy
- Periventricular leukomalacia (PVL) confirmed by neuroimaging (see section 2.2)
- Energy-inefficient gait
- Satisfactory muscle strength, generally defined as antigravity muscle strength at the hips and knees
- Fair or good selective motor control at the hips and knees, meaning the child should be able to partially isolate joint movement (not moving the joint in a patterned fashion), which requires sufficient strength and motor control (i.e., the child shouldn't be reliant on spasticity for their stability or movement)
- Good ability to cooperate with rehabilitation

Children who meet all the selection criteria are uncommon, so physicians use their judgment to determine whether a particular child is a good candidate for SDR.[228] Your team will assess whether SDR is suitable for your child based on their specific circumstances.

The thinking behind the ideal age of four to seven years for SDR is that gait is relatively stable, and it is possible to decrease spasticity while the child is still young enough to learn new motor patterns. As well, secondary contracture development is usually minimal at this point, and the child is old enough to complete the assessment and cooperate with the rigorous rehabilitation program. Gait analysis is very important for evaluating whether SDR is appropriate for a particular child and for assessing outcome after surgery. (Gait analysis is addressed in the next section.)

---

* Largely based on the work of Warwick Peacock, the neurosurgeon who repopularized and refined SDR in the 1980s and 1990s.

Children for whom SDR is not recommended include those with a predominance of dystonia, less severe spasticity, established contractures (typically in older children and adolescents), weakness, and poor selective motor control.[246] Though SDR is most effective in childhood, it is sometimes performed for adolescents and adults.

SDR reduces spasticity only. Any secondary problems—any muscle contractures and bone problems that are present—will remain after SDR. These may be treated by orthopedic surgery. SDR is for tone reduction; orthopedic surgery is for bone alignment and residual muscle tightness. In fact, it is important to note that as tone-reducing procedures, neither SDR nor ITB negates the need for orthopedic surgery—they are complementary procedures. The expectation should be that both tone reduction and orthopedic surgery may be needed. However, tone reduction can allow the orthopedic surgery to focus more on bone realignment than on tendon lengthening, as ROM frequently improves after SDR.

As with any treatment, prior goal-setting and being able to formally evaluate outcome is essential. SDR is a major operation, and the better the rehabilitation, the better the outcome is likely to be. Just as the operation itself varies between centers, so do post-SDR rehabilitation protocols. A review of post-SDR protocols found that patients undergo intensive PT lasting approximately one year starting in the first days after surgery. Patients remain hospitalized anywhere from six days to six weeks.[227]

As an example, at Gillette Children's, rehabilitation begins three days post-SDR and usually involves a four- to six-week hospital stay. The benefit of being an inpatient is that it allows for twice-daily therapy (PT, OT, and other therapies if necessary) and focuses on rehabilitation in this early postoperative period. Whether rehabilitation is inpatient or outpatient, the aim is to achieve the intensity of postoperative rehabilitation required to maximize functional outcomes. Information on rehabilitation after SDR at Gillette Children's is included in Appendix 6 (online).

Research supports SDR for reduced spasticity and improved gait (green light).[14] Studies of SDR showing improvements include both short- term and long-term studies (up to 26 years post-SDR).[228,247,248,249] Long-term follow-up of SDR indicates that over half the patients had orthopedic surgery in the follow-up years.[247,248] In their long-term follow-up study (10 to 17 years after SDR), Munger and colleagues reported that non-SDR patients had significantly more orthopedic surgery and antispasticity injections than SDR patients.[249] However, a multicenter study of long-term effects of SDR found that untreated spasticity does not cause meaningful impairments in young adulthood at the level of pathophysiology,[*] function, or quality of life.[250]

Choosing the tone-reducing treatment

No one treatment meets every child's needs, which is why a range of tone-reducing treatments exist. Tone reduction to manage spasticity (and dystonia, if present) is tailored to the individual child's needs. Which treatment will be recommended depends on many factors, including age, GMFCS level, degree to which the tone interferes with function, and type of high tone. A child may receive different treatments as they grow. For example, they may start with BoNT-A and then undergo SDR in later childhood when their gross motor function is more mature and their ability to participate in rehabilitation has improved.[228] Though the use of tone reduction peaks in early childhood, it can continue into adolescence and adulthood.

Some tone-reducing treatments (such as SDR and ITB) are available only at specialist centers. To be able to choose the most appropriate treatment for each individual child, access to the specialist center is needed to supplement what is available locally.

Finally, note that as with all areas in the management and treatment of CP, best practice may change as more research emerges.

---

* The study of how a condition affects the normal functioning of the body, leading to changes in its structure or function.

While SDR is mostly carried out on young children, it can be carried out on adults. Tommy had SDR as an adult in February 2020. While it was felt that it would not achieve any major gains in terms of gait, it would be protective of his muscles in the long term given his high level of spasticity. Unfortunately, February 2020 was just before the COVID-19 pandemic, which resulted in lack of access to rehabilitation.

Tommy

SDR surgery was the first major surgery I had that wasn't on one of my legs. On the one hand, spinal surgery is more serious, given the importance of the spinal cord. But from another perspective, it was just one incision, and given that I was able to be up and about relatively quickly, the recovery seemed easier.

The first part of the rehab involved lying entirely flat for 72 hours to let the area around the spinal cord heal. The spinal cord is surrounded by fluid, and the concern is that the fluid could leak from the incision with too much movement. This 72 hours of bed rest was quite boring, but the good folks at Mssrs. Netflix, Hulu, and Apple TV provided a lot of diversion. After the enforced bed rest, you start to come up to a sitting position gradually—my memory is of something like 10 degrees per hour over an afternoon. Sensation came back slowly to my feet, and it gave rise to the very strange feeling of all 10 of my toes individually against the blanket. "Legs!" I wrote to someone at the time. "I have legs! With feet! And so many toes!" From sitting, you can return fairly quickly to normal. I took my first steps with a walker three days post-op. The big concern during this time was falling, and so almost all of my walking was done with a loop around my chest that someone behind me could keep a hold of.

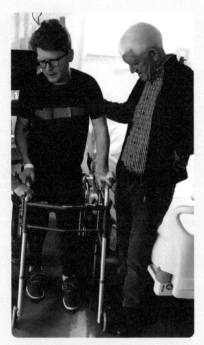

Tommy and his dad.

If possible, I recommend not doing the surgery in the middle of winter, but in true glass-half-full style, I just thought of the snow and ice outside the hospital as relearning how to walk on "hard mode." Relearning to walk was trippy, in both the literal and figurative senses of the word. I would struggle to send the correct signals from brain to feet: I'd try to move my foot two inches to the left and end up six inches out in front.

I stayed on crutches for about four weeks, as long as I was an outpatient at Gillette. I think I moved onto two crutches in part to not have to transport a walker on a plane back to San Francisco. I stayed using two crutches for probably another eight or nine months. COVID impacted my ability to see a physical therapist face-to-face, but as I write this three years later, I walk independently around the house or in the office, but otherwise use a crutch for uneven surfaces, long distances, or unfamiliar terrain. Three years on, I'm glad that I chose to do SDR (although, as I said, I recommend not doing so during winter, or before a global pandemic). I'm looser, with less spasticity and less tone. This presents itself in every-day life in ways such as being able to sit cross-legged for the first time as an adult. I'm also better able to bring my knees up to my chest, such as when sitting down and putting on socks. Somewhat strangely, I lost a lot of the ability to regulate temperature in my feet—they were very stiff and cold. I found it very uncomfortable to walk around barefoot, even just the short distance from the bedroom to the bathroom. My guess is that, since nerve endings do regulate temperature, my feet were having a harder time of this since 29 percent of those nerves were severed. With seemingly no explanation, this issue seems to have resolved itself three years on, and I can now walk around barefoot comfortably.

Orthopedic surgery

Fractures well cured make us more strong.

Ralph Waldo Emerson

There are two main peaks in the management of the musculoskeletal problems of spastic diplegia. The first occurs in early childhood, when tone reduction (in conjunction with other treatments such as PT and orthoses) is very important. The second occurs in later childhood (at approximately 8 to 12 years) when orthopedic surgery may be needed to address the secondary problems—the muscle and bone problems that have developed.[192]

Delaying orthopedic surgery allows motor patterns to mature, and by this stage the gains from tone reduction have largely been achieved. Delaying orthopedic surgery is also important because it helps avoid the unpredictable outcomes of early surgery[230] and recurrence of problems after surgery. Orthopedic surgery becomes necessary when the muscle and bone problems (the secondary problems) can no longer be adequately managed by more conservative means, and they are having a significant adverse effect on gait and function. Children at GMFCS level

III may reach the point of requiring orthopedic surgery earlier than children at lower GMFCS levels.

Single-event multilevel surgery (SEMLS) involves multiple orthopedic surgical procedures performed during a single operation. The goals are for the surgeon to identify and correct all the muscle and bone problems in the same surgery to avoid multiple hospital admissions, repeated anesthesia, and multiple rehabilitations. SEMLS is now considered best practice for orthopedic surgery in CP.[128]

This section addresses:

- **Three-dimensional gait analysis**
- **Single-event multilevel surgery**
- **Preserving plantar flexion strength**

Three-dimensional gait analysis

SEMLS in spastic diplegia is guided by computerized three-dimensional (3D) gait analysis,[74,141,251] which provides detailed information about a person's manner of walking and how far it deviates from typical walking. Computerized 3D gait analysis uses complex technology, some of it the same as what is used in the movie industry, such as in animations and video games. Gait analysis allows treatment to be individualized (i.e., tailored to each individual child), which is important because two children with spastic diplegia may walk in a similar manner, but the mechanisms behind their walking may differ. Analyzing those mechanisms prior to SEMLS is crucial for planning treatment.

Gait analysis is done for two main reasons:

- To identify all gait deviations and create a problem list. A treatment plan to meet the family's and surgeon's goals can then be devised. This is an example of data-driven decision-making in medicine.*
- To help measure the effectiveness of treatment—in other words, to assess the outcome of treatment. This allows for a critical appraisal

---

* Multiple variables are evaluated using multiple measurement tools within gait analysis.

of the decision-making process and the postoperative period (including rehabilitation) for the individual.

Analyzing gait is a complex process involving many technologies. The precise elements of gait analysis vary slightly between institutions. Gait analysis at Gillette Children's includes the following elements:[*]

- Medical history
- X-rays
- Parent-reported functional questionnaires for children (self-reported for older individuals where possible)
- Two-dimensional video
- Standardized physical examination
- 3D computerized motion analysis:[†]
  - Kinematics: 3D measurement of motion (movement)
  - Kinetics: 3D measurement of forces and mechanisms that cause motion
- Electromyography (EMG): measurement of the activity of muscles
- Pedobarography: measurement of the pressure distribution under the feet
- Energy expenditure: measurement of the energy used during walking

"Gait analysis," means including 3D computerized motion analysis. It does not mean merely observing gait or gait analysis done with simpler technologies. We acknowledge gait analysis is not universally available.

The key part of gait analysis is 3D computerized motion analysis, which measures gait in three planes simultaneously (hence the term "3D"). The three anatomical planes are illustrated in Figure 3.8.1. They are:

- From back or front: the coronal plane
- From the side: the sagittal plane
- From top or bottom: the transverse plane

---

[*] Some of these elements are also used at other times in the management of spastic diplegia, outside of formal gait analysis.

[†] 3D computerized motion analysis is the broader term because it includes other forms of motion besides gait, such as upper body motion. However, the terms "3D computerized motion analysis" and "3D computerized gait analysis" can be used interchangeably.

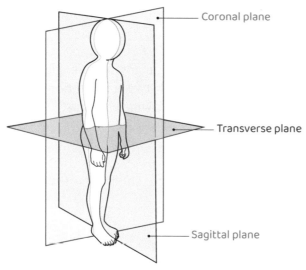

Figure 3.8.1 Anatomical planes.

The list of gait deviations is derived from the elements of gait analysis listed above. The information from all these sources provides a complete picture of a person's gait problems. Each source provides critical and unique information. When combined, data from one source can explain findings and/or complement data from another source. Comparing the gait of the individual with CP to a group of individuals with typical gait is very useful because it reveals how far the person's gait deviates from typical gait, as well as which joints are principally affected.

Once all the gait analysis data is collected, a team of professionals interprets all the pieces of data. This may include physicians, physical therapists, and engineers, all of whom have specialized training in this area. The team identifies gait deviations from the data, then creates a problem list from which a treatment plan can be devised. It is important to note that gait analysis provides only data; the *interpretation* of that data (i.e., to determine the gait deviations, problem list, and treatment plan) is done by the team of professionals. The family will typically meet their physician at a separate appointment to discuss the results.

I encourage all parents and people with the condition to obtain a copy of their gait report and read it. It is not a simple report by any means, but the explanations in this book will aid your understanding. Gait analysis is important when planning treatment. Given that parents and people with the condition are co-decision makers with professionals when planning treatment, a good understanding of the gait report is helpful in this role.

Repeat gait analysis after treatment is done to assess the treatment outcome. This closed-loop approach (plan, treat, evaluate) is very important for each individual because it objectively assesses whether the decisions and treatment (data interpretation, treatment plan, SEMLS, and rehabilitation) were effective and provides a new baseline for future comparison.

This closed loop leads to continuous improvement in the standard of treatment offered by a treatment center over the long term. For example, gait analysis can be used to evaluate the outcome of a group of children who had a particular procedure. Gait analysis may also be repeated many years after a procedure to evaluate the long-term outcome of that particular procedure. These evaluations inform practice at a center. In addition, shared learning and research lead to treatment improvements on a national and international level.

Reasons for referral for gait analysis vary between centers, but a referral is usually made when a person reaches a plateau in their progress and previous treatments are no longer effective. The age at which gait analysis is recommended varies, but it is usually recommended for children above three years of age, when gait is stable. Before age three, children are often too small, they are less able to tolerate the equipment and duration of the testing, and their walking pattern is still changing as it matures. When gait is changing, outcomes are less predictable. The ability to cooperate is also a consideration and is variable. It may remain challenging even in slightly older children.

Further information on gait analysis is included in Appendix 7 (online).

Single-event multilevel surgery

The number of procedures performed during SEMLS varies but could be as many as 8 to 16.[128] (A procedure is a single treatment for a muscle or bone. For example, lengthening of the gastrocnemius muscle is one procedure. If it is carried out on both legs, it counts as two procedures. A femoral derotation osteotomy is one procedure if it is carried out on one leg and two if it is carried out on both legs.) The number of procedures may seem overwhelming to the individual and family, but the purpose of the surgery is to correct all secondary problems in a single operation, so that a balance across all affected joints is achieved.

Before gait analysis was common, orthopedic surgery for children with CP typically involved doing single procedures on a yearly basis followed by intensive rehabilitation. Mercer Rang, an English-born orthopedic surgeon who practiced in Toronto, coined the phrase "birthday syndrome" to refer to this type of orthopedic surgery: the child had an operation each year, followed by rehabilitation for the rest of the year.[252] Thankfully, orthopedic surgery for CP has progressed significantly since those days.

As we have seen, many muscles span more than one joint. Thus, for example, a procedure at the ankle also affects the knee. A procedure at the knee also affects the hip and foot. This is another reason why SEMLS has replaced the "birthday syndrome" approach.

The overall goal of SEMLS is to improve or maintain gait over the long term. Secondary goals may include improvements in gait efficiency,* appearance, gross motor function, independence, and quality of life.[253] Improving gait efficiency might mean that the person doesn't tire as easily while walking, and improving the appearance of walking can have huge effects on self-esteem, particularly during adolescence.

The typical surgical team that performs SEMLS consists of two experienced surgeons with two assistants.[128] Having two surgical teams means one team can operate on one lower limb while the other operates on

---

* Gait efficiency can be measured by how much energy is consumed during walking. Think of energy expenditure during walking like the fuel efficiency of a car: a more efficient car will consume less fuel while traveling a set distance.

the other limb, minimizing the amount of time the patient spends under anesthesia.

Most care centers have patient education material that describes the different operations and what the individual and family can expect. Gillette Children's has developed a booklet, *All about Your Single-Event Multilevel Surgery (SEMLS)*, that explains possible procedures carried out as part of SEMLS. A link is included in **Useful web resources**.

Soft tissue surgery can include:

- **Tendon release:** Severing the tendon of a contracted muscle to allow for a greater range of motion of the joint. Once the tendon is severed, the function of the muscle is markedly diminished, which therefore decreases the problematic pull of the muscle.
- **Tendon transfer:** Reattaching the tendon at a different point to change the function of the muscle. For example, a muscle that behaved as a joint flexor, when transferred, could become a joint extensor. The goal is to improve the balance of muscles around a joint.
- **Muscle and/or tendon lengthening:** Lengthening the muscle and/or tendon, though not releasing the tendon entirely, allowing for continued action of that muscle.
- **Muscle recession:** Dividing the sheet of tissue where the muscle ends and the tendon begins. This is most commonly done in the calf, with the sheet of tissue of the gastrocnemius being separated from a similar sheet for the soleus (as they come together at their common Achilles tendon) and only the gastrocnemius tissue (the two-joint muscle) being divided.

It is important to note that with tendon release or muscle and/or tendon lengthening surgery, variable degrees of weakness occur, and with further growth, the contracture may recur.

The following are common soft tissue surgical procedures:

- Psoas lengthening
- Adductor lengthening
- Hamstring lengthening
- Rectus femoris transfer

- Calf muscle (gastrocnemius) lengthening/recession
- Tibialis anterior split transfer

Bone surgery can include:

- **Osteotomy:** Surgical cutting of a bone
- **Fusion:** Permanently joining two or more bones to eliminate joint movement and provide stability, also termed "arthrodesis"

The following are common bone surgical procedures:

- Pelvic osteotomy
- Proximal femoral osteotomy
- Distal femoral extension osteotomy
- Tibial tubercle/patella tendon advancement
- Tibial derotation osteotomy
- Various foot osteotomies and foot arthrodeses

As with all treatments, goal-setting is an important part of SEMLS. The expectations and goals of the surgeon and the family (both the parent and the child or adolescent) must be aligned and are part of shared decision-making in medical care. A recently developed outcome measure, the Gait Outcomes Assessment List (GOAL) questionnaire (two versions: one for the parent and one for the individual), evaluates family priorities in conjunction with gait-specific functional mobility outcomes.[187,188,189,190] It was developed with direct input from children with CP and their parents. Assessing priorities and goals on an item-by-item basis is useful because it can help the surgeon (or any care provider) understand the family's priorities and expectations and open a discussion about what can or cannot be achieved through surgery and subsequent rehabilitation. Ultimately, this results in a mutual understanding and alignment of goals for the proposed surgery.

We saw in Chapter 2 that three longitudinal studies found deterioration in gait over time in children and adolescents with untreated spastic diplegia.[143,144,145] The time interval for deterioration was as short as one and a half years. The aim of SEMLS is to counteract this deterioration and improve gait or maintain walking function. Because the natural history of gait in adolescence is of deterioration, even maintenance of gait should be viewed as success.

Although SEMLS is evidence-based best practice, Vuillermin and colleagues have noted that many orthopedic surgeons still perform single-level surgery because of differences in surgical philosophy as well as the limited availability of 3D gait analysis.[254]

SEMLS, like SDR, is usually followed by an intensive rehabilitation program to gain the maximum benefit from the surgery. The ultimate outcome is the result of the entire "package": the gait analysis–guided surgery planning, the surgical technique, and the postoperative rehabilitation. Family support systems also come into play. Most centers will consider SEMLS only if the child, with their family, is capable of completing the rehabilitation program. As with any orthopedic surgery, the better the rehabilitation, the better the outcome is likely to be.

The hospital stay for SEMLS is about two to four days. Though rehabilitation may begin with a hospital physical therapist, it is usually continued with the child's community physical therapist. Communication between hospital and community physical therapists is very important to ensure a smooth handover of care. Although there is no consensus on optimal rehabilitation post-SEMLS[255,256] work is being done to achieve this, and protocols have recently been developed.[256,257] Each person who undergoes SEMLS will receive a detailed rehabilitation program, which will vary depending on the procedures carried out during the surgery. Information on rehabilitation after SEMLS at Gillette Children's is included in Appendix 8 (online).

If implants (plates and/or screws inserted during surgery) are used in SEMLS, they may need to be removed approximately one year after surgery. The recovery from implant removal is minimal, and often the procedure does not require a hospital stay or any additional rehabilitation.

Following SEMLS, it typically takes nine months to a year for the child to return to their presurgical level of function (or longer, depending on age and other factors). Thus, full recovery following SEMLS can take up to one year, and the full benefit of surgery may not be seen for up to two years. Recovery is often longer in adolescents and adults compared to children. Short-term outcome after SEMLS including gait analysis is generally assessed when recovery is complete or nearly so (again, generally about one year after surgery).

Though SEMLS is a major undertaking, it should not be seen as an end point. It is just a treatment along the journey to adulthood for the child or adolescent with spastic diplegia. SEMLS cannot alter the primary problems (the underlying cause of impaired bone and muscle growth), and a gradual recurrence of some muscle and bone problems may occur post-SEMLS. Until the body reaches skeletal maturity, it is important to keep muscle growth at pace with continuing bone growth through activity, episodes of physical therapy, and consultation to update the home program. Puberty is a period of very active bone growth, so stretching and strengthening are as important in the years after SEMLS as they are in the years before.

Overall, there is good evidence supporting SEMLS.[251,253,255,258,259,260] The benefits include improvements in gait 12 months after surgery and improvements in gross motor function and quality of life 24 months after surgery.[253] Two longer-term studies—up to nine years after the original SEMLS—showed that the improvements were maintained.[251,259] However, in these studies, 39 percent[251] and 67 percent[259] of adolescents required additional orthopedic surgery (other than implant removal) in the years after their initial SEMLS. It should be noted, however, that the subsequent surgeries were less invasive (an average of two procedures, compared with eight to nine procedures for the original SEMLS) and required a shorter and easier period of rehabilitation.

It must be emphasized that SEMLS reduces, but does not eliminate, the possible need for further surgeries. Dreher and colleagues suggested the term "SEMLS" might be misleading because of the possibility of further surgery; they suggested removing "single-event" from the term and using "multilevel surgery (MLS)" for the initial surgery.[251] Regardless of the term used, the initial surgery is designed to correct muscle and bone problems in one surgical event. If further muscle and bone problems arise during subsequent adolescent growth, then further surgery may be required.

Our story refers to Gillette because that is where our son had SEMLS, but other specialist centers around the world offer this treatment. As with all treatments, different institutions and different providers may have different protocols.

In 2001, just after 9/11, Dr. Gage, an orthopedic surgeon at Gillette, presented at a conference I attended at the Central Remedial Clinic (CRC) in Dublin. That day I made a mental note that if Tommy ever needed orthopedic surgery, I would contact Dr. Gage. Unbeknownst to me, that day would arrive sooner than I realized. In 2003, orthopedic surgery was recommended for Tommy. I wrote to Dr. Gage, sending him Tommy's records (including his recent gait analysis, carried out at the CRC) and asking if he would be willing to see Tommy. We took Tommy to Minnesota to see Dr. Gage, who recommended SEMLS. To support my own understanding, I decided to complete a research master's: a case study providing a detailed picture of SEMLS and rehabilitation and evaluating outcome (up to two years post-SEMLS) using a comprehensive range of measurement tools.

My husband and I traveled from Ireland to Minnesota in 2004 with nine-year-old Tommy. Everyone at home was terribly worried about us taking Tommy abroad for orthopedic surgery. Neither professionals nor friends supported our decision. The most support we had was from our family physician, who said the amount of surgery the SEMLS would entail was akin to a very bad road traffic accident, but at least the surgery would be planned and they would not be picking glass fragments from Tommy's muscle tissue. Positive, but not exactly a ringing endorsement! And those were the only words of "encouragement" we heard amid a lot of well-meaning discouragement, including, "They cut too much in America."

Despite all the worry and lack of support back home, we—Tommy, my husband, and I—were not at all worried. We had complete confidence in Dr. Gage and the surgical team at Gillette.

In writing this book I have reflected on why I felt so confident in our decision to pursue SEMLS despite the negative reactions of so many people, including many for whom I had and still have a huge amount of respect. It really came down to this:

- The explanation of the primary, secondary, and tertiary problems in spastic diplegia was logical, as was the logic of the treatment plan.
- I understood that SEMLS required pediatric orthopedists who were specialists in analyzing gait in CP and well versed in 3D computerized motion analysis, that planning this type of orthopedic surgery was not like planning a knee or hip replacement, and that the complexity and skill involved in the surgery lay in the choice of which procedures to perform. I recognized that Gillette had developed this expertise.
- At that time (2004), SEMLS was supported by research from a number of international centers.[98,261-264] An early 2001 research study from Gillette[98] was followed by a more detailed study in early 2004,[263] just prior to Tommy's SEMLS. The 2004 outcome study included 66 patients with an average age of nine with a diagnosis of spastic diplegia and no prior surgical procedure—exactly the same as Tommy. This study showed that gait pattern, gait efficiency (energy consumed while walking), community walking, and higher-level functional skills improved after orthopedic surgery for the majority of those patients. (Since that time, studies from many international centers have supported SEMLS, including the first randomized controlled trial of SEMLS in CP.)[253]
- The attitude of humility, care, and respect for children with CP at Gillette was extraordinary. I have visited a number of times in the intervening years and this still hits me every single time. The combination of world-class expertise and world-class care is amazing.

Tommy's operation lasted six hours. He had 13 procedures in all, 9 on his right leg and 4 on his left. Despite all the procedures, he refused to take any pain medication once he left the hospital four days later. (Having left the hospital, his only "medication" if he woke in pain during the night was having his dad sing him back to sleep or watching videos.)

An intensive, year-long rehabilitation back in Ireland (based on Gillette's rehabilitation plan) followed the surgery. No one should underestimate the amount and intensity of rehabilitation required after SEMLS: it took a lot of work on Tommy's (and our) part. Rehabilitation after SEMLS is a lot longer than rehabilitation following, say, knee replacement surgery.

I would advise each individual and parent to understand what they are signing up for when they plan to undergo SEMLS. Surgery is only the start of a long road. In a sense, once you've driven away from the hospital following the surgery, the hard work (for the child and the parent) is only just beginning. However, the long rehabilitation will likely be very much worth it.

Surgery can be regarded as a three-part process: good surgical planning, good surgery, and good rehabilitation. The surgeon is responsible for the first two parts, and the parent and child, in conjunction with the physical therapist, are largely responsible for the third. A successful outcome requires all three.

We stayed in the US for six weeks. Ideally, SEMLS and the period immediately following discharge from the hospital require the support of two adults; in my opinion it is too much work for just one. The surgery wasn't easy for Tommy, nor for us. It was difficult leaving our other children at home and being away for so long. But without a shadow of a doubt, we would do it all again.

Rehabilitation from SEMLS can take up to one year, and the full benefit of the surgery may not be seen for up to two years. I remember how surprised people were to see how much less functional Tommy was after his SEMLS. Without understanding what was involved, they expected to see near-immediate improvements. Tommy had his implants (the plates and screws inserted during surgery) removed in Dublin one year later.

In my research study, SEMLS was judged to have been successful by all stakeholders (child, parent, surgeon, and teacher). Objective measures of change included improvements in gait, endurance, gross motor function, muscle strength, and flexibility. Patient and parent satisfaction were evident in interviews conducted by my research supervisor with Tommy and his dad. One of the most noticeable findings from the interviews with Tommy was how unconcerned he was about the surgery, both before and after, and how positive his outlook was throughout. (To keep his mind off surgery and later as pain medication, we used distraction techniques: Tommy had asked for a particular box set of videos, which we bought but didn't allow him to start watching until he was in the hospital. As a result, he couldn't wait to get to the hospital. Heading to the operating room on the morning of the surgery, he wasn't anxious; he was just disappointed he had to press pause on the DVD player.)

Once we made the decision to proceed with SEMLS in the US, the staff at the CRC and our community physical therapist could not have been more helpful. They provided information to the team in the US in advance, stayed in touch with us while we were away, and supported Tommy's long rehabilitation afterward. In addition, the CRC gait lab and our community physical therapist provided data and other assistance to help me complete my master's.

When Tommy was 16 years old, he developed severe knee pain. He has a high pain threshold, but the pain was so bad that it interfered with his sleep. We tried a number of treatments without success. We contacted the surgeons at Gillette, who immediately recognized the cause and advised further orthopedic surgery. Tommy had two additional orthopedic surgeries when he was 16 and 18. By this time, Dr. Gage had retired and Dr. Novacheck was at the helm. Tommy's surgery at age 16 included five procedures on his right leg to address the knee pain and other issues that had arisen during adolescence. The later surgery, at age 18, was an adjustment to one of the earlier procedures.

His surgery at age 18 coincided with a cycling trip through France my husband and I had planned for our 25th wedding anniversary. Our three sons insisted the cycling trip continue, and the older boys, now living in the US, decided they would accompany Tommy to the surgery. While I wanted to postpone the trip, I was totally outnumbered by the men in my life. In the end, we took the cycling trip, and I felt relaxed and not at all worried because of my confidence in Dr. Novacheck and our three boys.

Based on our journey and everything I have read, I can honestly say Tommy would not be walking as well or living as independently as he is today without the surgeries he had in his adolescent years. In the early days, we had been told that Tommy would likely need to use a wheelchair by the time he was in college. I mentioned earlier that my favorite photograph from Tommy's graduation is a shot of him and the family walking to dinner that evening, and that I felt compelled to send a copy of it to the many professionals who helped Tommy reach that day.

Indeed, in 2023, Tommy, himself, sent his wedding photo to the same group.

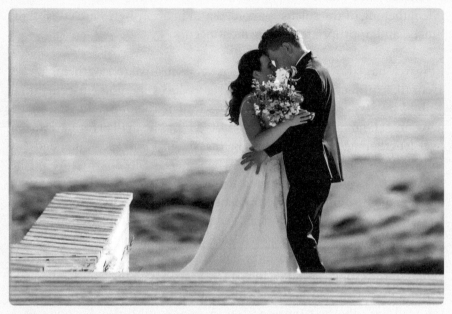

Tommy and Lindsey. Photo by Nicole Goddard Photography, Inc.

Preserving plantar flexor strength

There is one important last point before leaving orthopedic surgery. In section 2.9, we saw that any treatment that weakens the ankle plantar flexors (the soleus and gastrocnemius–the calf muscles) may contribute to crouch gait.[128] Therefore, preserving plantar flexion strength is *key* for preventing crouch gait.

In a study of the prevalence of severe crouch gait over a 15-year period, severe crouch gait was found to be precipitated by lengthening of either the Achilles tendon or the gastrocnemius and soleus in combination* that was not part of SEMLS.[254] This is consistent with earlier studies,[265,266] which found that the majority of those who develop more severe crouch

---

* The Achilles tendon is common to both the gastrocnemius and soleus muscles. The lengthening of the soleus and gastrocnemius in combination is performed closer to where the muscles join the tendon but still includes both muscles.

gait had previous Achilles tendon lengthening. It may be necessary to lengthen the short two-joint gastrocnemius, but the single-joint soleus is generally not short.[128] It appears severe crouch can largely be avoided if lengthening of the soleus is avoided and in a setting where consistent, timely, and appropriate management occurs.

Research has shown that the soleus is very sensitive to lengthening.[267] A 1 cm (0.4 in) lengthening of the soleus reduces its moment-generating ability* by 50 percent, and a 2 cm (0.8 in) lengthening reduces it by 85 percent.[268] Graham and colleagues noted that "a small error in terms of over-lengthening the soleus may be disastrous" and recommended "to lengthen the gastrocnemius only, when there is no contracture in the soleus."[128] They further reported that there is usually a delay between this lengthening and the development of crouch gait: the lengthening is often done between three and six years of age, and it may take another three to six years before crouch gait becomes a significant problem. It may only be when the adolescent growth spurt occurs that the full extent of the crouch gait develops. (The reason why the lengthening was commonly performed between three and six years of age was because toe walking—the first pattern seen in spastic diplegia—becomes very prevalent at that age.[139] The lengthening was to address toe walking. Toe walking is a noticeable gait deviation and an unstable form of walking.)

If there is muscular contracture in the calf, in spastic diplegia, the gastrocnemius is essentially always much more contracted than the soleus. If there is soleus contracture, it should be managed as conservatively as possible. Graham and colleagues recommend that when the soleus requires lengthening it should only be done using a very precise and stable technique.[128] Lengthening of the Achilles tendon in effect lengthens both muscles, and therefore it will likely overlengthen and weaken the soleus muscle. In addition, while percutaneous lengthening surgery† (surgery done through the skin, often referred to as "percs" or "selective percutaneous myofascial lengthening" [SPML]) may be easier on the child than traditional surgery, the surgery is performed at the level of the Achilles tendon. Consensus exists that surgery performed at the level of the Achilles tendon should be avoided in spastic diplegia.[269]

---

* See section 2.4. for explanation of "moment."

† Percutaneous lengthening surgery can be done to other muscle-tendon units, not just the calf muscles and Achilles tendon.

Thankfully, nowadays surgeons usually lengthen the gastrocnemius alone, but I caution readers that the old procedure may still be carried out in some parts of the world and at less specialized institutions. I encourage readers to always understand what lengthening is being done if surgery for the calf muscles (the gastrocnemius and soleus) is being proposed. It is important to know which muscle is being lengthened.

Be especially careful about percutaneous lengthening of calf muscles.

Managing associated problems

The purpose of life is to live it, to taste experience to the utmost, to reach out eagerly and without fear for newer and richer experience.

Eleanor Roosevelt

We saw in sections 2.1 and 2.10 that a proportion of children with spastic diplegia (all GMFCS levels) have associated problems. The management of each of these challenges needs to be addressed as part of the multidisciplinary care of the child and adolescent with spastic diplegia. These problems, if present and unaddressed or inadequately addressed, may reduce participation far more than their musculoskeletal/mobility problems.

- **Speech, language and communication, and feeding:** The management of speech, language and communication, and feeding was addressed in section 3.4.
- **Sensory problems:** Sensory problems are primary problems and are more difficult to remediate. Early intervention that taps into neuroplasticity can help.
- **Vision:** For those with vision challenges, an early referral to a pediatric ophthalmologist and regular follow-up is important. Pediatric

ophthalmologists specialize in concerns related to vision and eye health for children. These specialists are medical doctors. An optometrist can evaluate for some concerns with vision, but they are not trained to do surgery on the eyes. Vision development is rapid from birth to age six but visual acuity (sharpness) can continue to change throughout life. If any concerns are noted, annual follow-up with pediatric ophthalmology is recommended.

- **Hearing:** Early screening for hearing loss should be done, as hearing loss can impact the development of speech, language, and communication, and cognition. Hearing loss can be difficult to evaluate in an individual with cognitive problems; however, specialized testing is available for those unable to recognize and reliably respond to sounds. Early referral to an audiologist, an otolaryngologist (a physician specializing in ear, nose, and throat, or ENT), and a speech-language pathologist is recommended if there is any hearing loss. Regular follow-up will be necessary. As with vision, once hearing problems are identified, supports can be determined for the child to enjoy maximum participation.

- **Epilepsy:** For those with epilepsy, regular and routine evaluation and follow-up with pediatric neurology is imperative as untreated epilepsy has the potential to slow or cause regression in development. Furthermore, although seizures are often thought of as being obvious abnormal movements that persist and are therefore unmistakable as epilepsy, seizures can be very quiet and challenging to identify, or even occur without any outward signs. Close surveillance by neurology specialists is required if there are any concerns related to seizure activity. Intervening to address seizure activity can allow the child to make significant gains in their development once the abnormal brain activity has been stopped. More information on epilepsy management is included in Appendix 9 (online).

- **Pain:** Because pain is prevalent in CP, the presence of pain should be closely monitored and addressed throughout childhood and adolescence. Early recognition of pain is important because pain in children with CP significantly reduces quality of life and is connected to mental health.[151] When pain is severe and prolonged, involving a specialist in pain should be considered. Pain specialists focus on alleviating pain using a multimodal approach, frequently combining nonmedication modalities with medications to maximize relief and improve comfort. It is important to support children with language about pain (e.g., how to describe pain) and how to advocate for their needs, not just accept that their pain is normal.

- **Nutrition and hydration:** Good nutrition and hydration are as important for the child and adolescent with spastic diplegia as they are for their peers. No special diet is needed so long as they are eating a nutritious, balanced diet. Parents are encouraged to get advice on this if necessary; the whole family might benefit. One area affected by nutrition is bone health. As shown in section 2.7, there is some evidence of lower bone mineral density in ambulatory children (and adults) with CP GMFCS levels II and III.[270] To promote optimum bone health throughout life, good nutrition, ensuring no deficiencies in calcium and vitamin D, and physical activity, especially weight-bearing or impact activities, can help promote good bone health.[271] It is also worth noting that some medications, for example, antiseizure medications and steroids, may contribute to lower bone mineral density. Weight management is also important; it's important for everyone, but even more so for people with spastic diplegia because muscle strength is already compromised, and excess weight can limit walking.[272] Good eating habits start early in life, and children are much more likely to have good habits if their parents do. The influence of parents can have an impact long after the child has left home. It is never too late to recognize unhealthy eating habits and make the decision to change.

- **Urinary and bowel continence:** A US study reported that 90 percent of individuals with spastic diplegia and quadriplegia (all GMFCS levels) who had symptomatic neurogenic bladder (SNB) achieved continence by nonsurgical care.[91] Treatment included a functional toileting review and medication. Urinary continence was found to be related to ability to communicate and environmental opportunity to succeed.

- **Constipation:** Constipation should be closely monitored throughout childhood and adolescence and addressed if present. It can contribute to pain and can complicate toilet training and contribute to urinary incontinence.

- **Sleep:** Because one-third of ambulatory children with CP have disturbed sleep[149] and sleep is required for good daytime function and development, sleep quality should be closely monitored throughout childhood and adolescence, and any problems should be addressed. A healthy nighttime routine is encouraged to promote good sleep. This includes limiting screen time (no screens 60 minutes before bedtime) and keeping screens and other distractions out of the bedroom. Choosing a regular bedtime that allows for adequate sleep through the night, and sticking to it nightly, promotes healthy sleep patterns. These efforts are collectively referred to as "sleep hygiene." If the child is having trouble falling asleep or staying asleep despite good sleep hygiene, their physician should be consulted.

- **Cognition:** Two in five children with spastic diplegia have some level of intellectual challenge,[80] so close attention should be paid to how well the child is learning from very early in life. By the time the child is preparing to move into kindergarten, elementary, or primary school, definitive neuropsychological testing* may be considered. This formal evaluation of the brain's processing of information allows the child, the family, and the school team to identify where there may be challenges in learning, and to gain understanding of how the child learns best. This allows for the teaching team to adapt the learning environment to maximize the child's ability for success. Adequate support in school needs to be addressed both from a cognitive and social perspective. The earlier challenges can be identified, the sooner the child can receive support services to maximize their function. The wider aspects of education are addressed in section 3.11.

- **Sexual relationships:** This is an area where both the family and professional team can support the adolescent with CP. Despite data showing that young adults with CP may experience problems with sexual relationships, 90 percent reported not having discussed the topic with health care professionals.[156] Health care professionals need to be proactive to inform young people with CP about sexual relationships to prevent sexual difficulties and to treat problems if they arise.[156]

- **Mental and behavioral health:** Mental and behavioral health symptoms and disorders are common in children and adolescents with CP.[159,160] Evaluations for mental and behavioral health should be incorporated into multidisciplinary assessments for individuals with CP, and appropriate treatments prescribed. Treatments for mental and behavioral health disorders are similar to those for typically developing children and adolescents and may include behavioral

---

* Neuropsychological testing helps evaluate broad areas of cognitive function; for example, intelligence, language, visuospatial function, executive function, attention, memory and processing speed. These areas frequently work in collaboration for efficient cognitive functioning.

therapy, psychotherapy, and medications.[162] Parenting programs that help parents manage challenging behavior may be of help. There is evidence supporting the Stepping Stones Triple P program for improving child behavior and reducing parental stress (green light).[14] This program, specifically for parents of preadolescent children who have a disability, is available online, and a link to its website is included in **Useful web resources.**

Alternative and complementary treatments

It is possible in medicine, even when you intend to do good, to do harm instead. That is why science thrives on actively encouraging criticism rather than stifling it.

Richard Dawkins

Alternative (as a substitute) and complementary (in addition to) treatments are treatments that are not part of current standard conventional medical or rehabilitation treatments and care.[273]

Parents want only the best for their children, and for a number of reasons they may consider alternative and complementary treatments. These reasons can include:

- Hearing about a treatment option in the media (Internet, radio, TV, newspapers, magazines) or from well-meaning family and friends
- Wanting to try all treatment options in case the one they haven't tried is the one that works
- Wanting to complement or increase the effectiveness of present treatment

- Wanting to relieve symptoms (such as pain)
- Believing their child can do better

Often, alternative and complementary treatments are expensive. If the parent-professional relationship is good, parents should be able to discuss them with the medical professionals who treat their child. Both parents and professionals should be guided by the best research evidence available, which is the very principle that has guided the writing of this book.

Table 3.10.1 lists a number of common alternative and complementary treatments.

Table 3.10.1 Alternative and complementary treatments

TREATMENT	DESCRIPTION	EVIDENCE (OR LACK OF) SUPPORTING TREATMENT IN CP
Hyperbaric oxygen	The person inhales 100 percent oxygen in a pressurized hyperbaric chamber. The theory behind its use in CP is that there are inactive cells among the damaged brain cells that have the potential to recover.	Strong recommendation against its use for all purposes (red light).*[14]
Massage	Involves applying pressure to muscles, generally using the hands, to relieve pain and tension.	Green light for improved passage of stool frequency. Yellow light for other purposes.[14]
Osteopathy (including cranial sacral osteopathy)	Treatment through the manipulation and massage of skeleton and muscles. Cranial sacral osteopathy focuses on the cranium (bones of the skull) and sacrum (the five fused vertebrae that connect the spine to the pelvis).	Strong recommendation against its use (red light) for improved gross motor function. Yellow light for reduced constipation and improved sleep.[14]
Acupuncture	Thin needles are inserted into the skin at specific points.	Yellow light for improved gross motor function and reduced spasticity.[14]

* See section 3.3 for explanation of traffic light system.[14]   *Cont'd.*

TREATMENT	DESCRIPTION	EVIDENCE (OR LACK OF) SUPPORTING TREATMENT IN CP
Reflexology	Massage based on the theory that there are reflex points on the feet, hands, and head linked to every part of the body.	Yellow light for reduced spasticity, improved gross motor function, and reduced constipation.[14]
Yoga	A practice that includes specific body postures, breath control and meditation.	Yellow light for multiple outcomes.[14]

Novak and colleagues' summary of the state of the evidence as of 2019 for interventions for children with CP (including further alternative and complementary treatments),[14] is included in **Useful web resources.**

A Canadian study looked at the extent to which adolescents with CP across all five GMFCS levels had used alternative and complementary treatments in the previous year. The most commonly used were massage (15 percent), hyperbaric oxygen (10 percent), and osteopathy (6 percent), but most of those surveyed (73 percent) did not currently use any.[273]

Graham noted that many parents delay or refuse conventional treatments because they have unrealistic expectations of other unproven treatments. For example, although Australia has an efficient hip surveillance program, the most common cause of a dislocated hip in a child with CP is delayed intervention because they have heard that stem cell treatment* may cure the child.[274]

Parents cannot afford to abandon conventional treatments with their evidence base for any unproven treatment, nor should they delay care that is currently available for their child, anticipating that a better option is "around the corner." As treatments are studied and when they are identified as potentially helpful, good physicians will be aware of the developing research and will share with families if any new options are on the horizon.

---

* An alternative treatment that may potentially replace damaged nerve cells and support remaining ones in the brain.

Community integration, education, independence, and transition

The Child is father of the Man.
William Wordsworth

Going through the normal changes of puberty, graduating from high school, choosing the next life stage, leaving home, assuming responsibility for one's own health care, and transitioning from the familiar and more organized setting of children's health services to the unfamiliar and more fragmented adult services—putting it all together, there is a lot going on packed into a short amount of time in the life of a child and adolescent with spastic diplegia.

A study of older adolescents with CP (age 18 to 20) defined success in life as being happy. Three key psychosocial factors related to this success were being believed in, believing in oneself, and being accepted by others (a sense of belonging).[275] The seeds of these factors are sown early in life, and parents do the sowing—through supporting community integration, education, independence, and transition.

Drs. Rosenbaum and Rosenbloom give some excellent advice to parents to take the long view when it comes to the life of the child with CP and supporting them into adulthood:[8]

> We encourage [parents] to take a long-term view of their child's journey through childhood. We remind them that the adult world imposes on all children the expectation (at least in school) that they try to perform in a wide range of areas. Adults expect children to learn and hopefully demonstrate skills in many activities—be they social, physical, intellectual, artistic—that are much more demanding than what the adults ever expect of themselves, or even perform, on a day-to-day basis ... [Parents] can help their children weather the childhood years with these many and varied demands (demands which often challenge many children without disabilities) ... in the course of their developing years, to develop competencies, interests, and a sense of self-confidence despite their "disabilities," because after the childhood years they will have many more opportunities to find their niche in life.

Community integration

The diagnosis of CP typically occurs early in life when the nuclear family—parents and siblings—play a large part in the infant's life. However, as the child grows, their social circle expands. It is important for all children, regardless of disability, to be integrated into their communities. In section 1.8, we addressed the ICF framework, which provides an understanding of how a health condition affects individuals across various levels and their interconnectedness. This framework underscores the importance of considering the broader context in which a person with a disability exists, aiming for their full participation in the community. Both environmental and personal factors exert influence at every level within the framework.

It is important to recognize that having a disability does not define a person, whether they are a child, adolescent, or adult. The family's perception and treatment of a child with a disability are critical, as they set the tone for how others, including extended family, friends, and teachers, will view and interact with the child. It is essential for the family to avoid perceiving the child as more limited than they actually are and, rather, foster an environment that encourages the child's full potential. A simple way to check yourself on this is to think about how you, the parent, assign chores and responsibilities to a typically developing child and then modify that task as needed and assign it to the child with CP. This supports their active role in the family and later independence.

Self-determination refers to a person's ability to act as their own primary decision maker. Independent of cognitive level, young adults with disabilities who demonstrate increased levels of self-determination have been found to fare better across multiple life categories, including employment, access to health care and other benefits, financial independence, and independent living.[276] It is also useful to instill an aptitude for self-advocacy—the ability to represent oneself or one's views or interests.

As social beings, humans require social connections for optimal mental health and well-being throughout their lives. Building strong social connections is crucial, and any factors that enhance social connectedness are valuable. Engaging in exercise and physical activities can be an excellent means to promote community integration. These activities can be pursued with the family and alongside nondisabled friends in informal settings rather than in therapy settings. In fact, the child's need for physical exercise can motivate the entire family to become more active. Choosing activities that are enjoyable for both the child and the family increases the likelihood that everyone will stick with it.

Tom Shakespeare, a prominent disability rights activist in the UK, argues that social barriers often pose more significant challenges than the impairments themselves. These barriers include lack of access and negative attitudes.

Education

Damiano considered physical activity to be very important in CP—titling a paper "Activity, Activity, Activity: Rethinking Our Physical Therapy Approach to Cerebral Palsy."[277] A further mantra could be "Education, Education, Education." A person with a physical challenge is less likely to choose employment in a role requiring significant physical prowess; they will more likely rely on other skills. It is important to maximize the child's intellectual abilities to maximize their opportunities for employment and their participation in all aspects of life. A good education is important for every child—indeed, education is included in the United Nations Convention on the Rights of the Child.[278] And a good education is needed to open doors to different careers. Today, the range of career options available to people with spastic diplegia is large; their disability places only a small limit on their choice.

Given that teachers have such a profound influence on the lives of their students, parents should speak with their child's teacher to ensure they understand both the child's abilities and their challenges. This is not a one-off conversation—as the child progresses through school, teachers change. If the student has multiple teachers, talking with a key staff member may work best.

We saw in section 2.1 that most children with spastic diplegia across all GMFCS levels have no intellectual problems, but a small percentage (15 percent) have moderate to severe intellectual problems.[80] Careful planning at each stage of school is needed to maximize the school experience of children and adolescents with intellectual problems. This will ensure sufficient accommodations are made to ease transitions and optimize the child's opportunity for a good education.

Health care professionals can be a good resource for planning ahead and problem-solving if or when challenges arise. Practicing skills that might be needed in the next phase of life at home with time, supervision, and someone with whom to problem-solve is highly beneficial, both for activity completion and to boost the child's self-confidence. One example is practicing dressing skills for changing in the locker room.

Regrettably, school bullying continues to affect significant numbers of children and adolescents, and those with disabilities are at higher risk.[279] One study found that children and adolescents with CP experienced bullying and social exclusion at school.[161] Strategies suggested by the children and adolescents to help improve social inclusion at school include:[280]

- Creating awareness of their disability by disclosing their condition to peers and teachers (with the suggestion that health care professionals could help with this)

- Being vocal about incidents of bullying and exclusion (to peers, teachers, and parents)
- Building quality friendships as an effective peer support network

They also emphasized the importance of teachers paying close attention to the needs of students with disabilities. A student teacher who has mild CP created the following excellent tip sheet for teachers of students with mild CP.[281] (A link to the full paper is included in **Useful web resources.**)

- There are varying forms of CP. CP can involve just physical symptoms, but it may be accompanied by intellectual or learning disabilities.
- Many students have surgery when young and may be in casts or use wheelchairs following surgery and will need extra support during this time.
- Students may become fatigued due to the extra physical strain involved in carrying out everyday tasks, such as writing, walking, or playing at recess.
- Most students experience pain at some point in the day, although they will be used to it and may not mention it.
- Most students with CP want to be treated like other students, so they may not ask for help when they need it.
- Most students with mild CP do not want attention drawn to them because of their disability.
- Teachers should be attentive to students' hesitation to participate in physical activities they may feel uncomfortable with.
- Teachers should intervene when young children ask questions that appear insensitive or call children with CP inappropriate names.
- When students talk about their CP, do not express sympathy; it is a part of who they are.

Social support for children struggling to connect with their peers may be available through the child's school team. Assertively pursuing these connections for the child who is struggling is imperative so that they may feel integrated into their social school environment. Social engagement goals could also be built into occupational and speech therapy.

Change is the one constant in life. Transitions are a big step for any child, and they keep coming: from home to daycare, to preschool, to elementary school, middle school, high school, and on to college, higher education, or work. Transitions can be more challenging for the child with CP because of, for example, difficulties with mobility or difficulties participating in some activities at school.

Independence

When does adolescence actually begin? The World Health Organization defines adolescence as the period between 10 and 19 years of age. The great majority of adolescents are, therefore, included in the age-based definition of the child adopted by the UN Convention on the Rights of the Child, which defines a child as a person under age 18.[278] Adolescence can thus be viewed as that vaguely defined period between childhood and adulthood. The adolescent is gaining independence from the parent but is not yet there.

For children with moderate to severe intellectual problems, independence in adulthood may not be a realistic goal. Questions such as legal guardianship, supported living arrangements, and shared decision-making will need to be considered. For where independence is a realistic goal, there are points to consider.

Parents play a huge role in the life of their child, and assuming the child achieves independence, a much smaller role in the life of their adult son or daughter. At some point in adolescence, we parents must try to facilitate this change. This is a change for both the parent and the adolescent, and it ideally happens gradually, over time. Indeed, increasing independence ought to begin early in childhood: we need to be preparing for this separation from the cradle.

The parent has to learn to cut the cord at the end of adolescence, but the adolescent also has to be ready for the cord to be cut: it is a two-way process. As with exercise and good eating habits, the foundations for becoming an independent adult are laid early in childhood.

Leaving the security of home is daunting for any adolescent, and they need to be equipped with the skills to look after themselves. The adolescent with spastic diplegia also needs to be able to manage their own health care as much as possible. Health care for the person with spastic diplegia usually changes from pediatric to adult services at the end of adolescence, which is another daunting change. It can be a big challenge for an adolescent to lose the services from professionals that they have effectively grown up with.

Being able to practice independence in a safe environment is important. For example, the adolescent can start running their own medical appointments with a parent there as a safety net and support, or complete chores or cook at home with the parent there to help if something goes wrong. In the age of increasingly digital communication, it can be helpful for the adolescent to be involved in phone conversations that they will be responsible for as they age. Using a speaker phone to include the young person when scheduling appointments or resolving issues with, for example, payment of services can be helpful. Initially the adolescent can listen, but over time, the parent can listen and coach. Practicing these skills at home, in a familiar environment, and learning from mistakes in a safe setting makes the transition to their highest level of independence less difficult, less scary, and more successful. Occupational therapy is a great resource in this area.

Thomason and Graham made the very interesting point that the decision to proceed with SEMLS for younger children is largely made by parents, but adolescents must be given the freedom to make their own informed decisions about surgery and rehabilitation.[282] They added that an adolescent who feels they have been forced into SEMLS against their will or without their full consent is likely to be resentful and may develop depression and struggle with rehabilitation. Indeed, this advice may be applicable to other areas in the life of the adolescent.

It's important to remember that the road to independence starts early in life. Then, the child is too young to participate in education around diagnosis, cause, and expectations for the future. However, families need to actively pass on this education to the child at age-appropriate times in their life to prepare them for living with their condition in adulthood. Too often, older children, adolescents, and adults have little understanding of their condition, which can hamper their involvement in management of their condition and independence.

Transition

Health care transition is defined as the planned process and skill-building to empower adolescents and their families to navigate an adult model of health care. It is more than simply changing medical professionals (termed "transfer").

Pediatric services for CP care are usually much better resourced than adult services and are better at following up with the individual. With adult services for CP care, it is usually up to the individual and family to do more proactive service procuring. Adult services are often much more reactionary rather than proactive.

Transition involves three steps: preparing, transferring, and integrating into adult services. That is, just because a file has been transferred does not mean the individual has successfully integrated into an adult service provider.

Helping children and adolescents with spastic diplegia to become as independent as possible is the overall goal, which is why the focus on that transition must start early (from about the age of 12)—although supporting their independence really starts from birth. Transition doesn't involve just health care; it also involves other areas such as education, finance, insurance coverage, and guardianship planning. It is very important that the individual with CP is involved.

Figure 3.11.1 is a comprehensive look at some important transition questions the individual needs to ask: Where will I live? Who is my care team? How will I pay for things? What will I do?

Figure 3.11.2 shows a typical form that can be used for preparing an individual for transition to adult services.

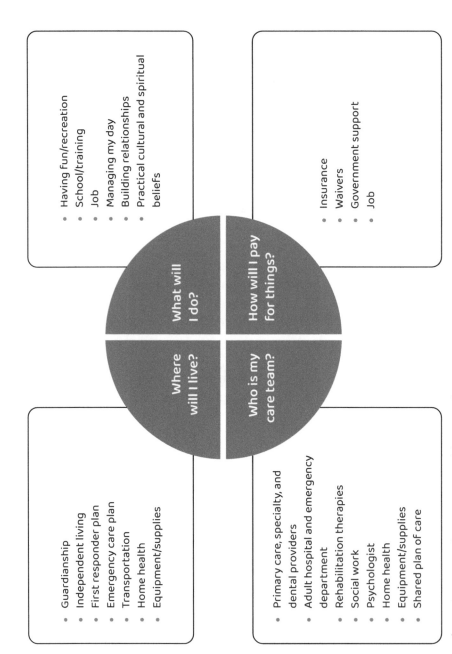

- Having Fun/recreation
- School/training
- Job
- Managing my day
- Building relationships
- Practical cultural and spiritual beliefs

- Insurance
- Waivers
- Government support
- Job

What will I do?

How will I pay for things?

Where will I live?

Who is my care team?

- Guardianship
- Independent living
- First responder plan
- Emergency care plan
- Transportation
- Home health
- Equipment/supplies

- Primary care, specialty, and dental providers
- Adult hospital and emergency department
- Rehabilitation therapies
- Social work
- Psychologist
- Home health
- Equipment/supplies
- Shared plan of care

Figure 3.11.1 Some important transition questions.

Transition Readiness Assessment Questionnaire (TRAQ)

Patient Name: _____ Date of Birth: ___/___/___ Today's Date ___/___/___ (MRN#_____)

**Directions to Youth and Young Adults:** Please check the box that best describes _your_ skill level in the following areas that are important for transition to adult health care. There is no right or wrong answer and your answers will remain confidential and private.
**Directions to Caregivers/Parents:** If your youth or young adult is unable to complete the tasks below on their own, please check the box that best describes _your_ skill level. **Check here** if you are a parent/caregiver completing this form. ☐

	No, I do not know how	No, but I want to learn	No, but I am learning to do this	Yes, I have started doing this	Yes, I always do this when I need to
Managing Medications					
1. Do you fill a prescription if you need to?					
2. Do you know what to do if you are having a bad reaction to your medications?					
3. Do you reorder medications before they run out?					
4. Do you explain any medications (name and dose) you are taking to healthcare providers?					
5. Do you speak with the pharmacist about drug interactions or other concerns related to your medications?					
Appointment Keeping					
6. Do you call the doctor's office to make an appointment?					
7. Do you follow-up on referrals for tests or check-ups or labs?					
8. Do you arrange for your ride to medical appointments?					
9. Do you call the doctor about unusual changes in your health (for example: allergic reactions)?					
Tracking Health Issues					
10. Do you fill out the medical history form, including a list of your allergies?					
11. Do you keep a calendar or list of medical and other appointments?					
12. Do you tell the doctor or nurse what you are feeling?					
13. Do you contact the doctor when you have a health concern?					
14. Do you make or help make medical decisions pertaining to your health?					
15. Do you attend your medical appointment or part of your appointment by yourself?					
Talking with Providers					
16. Do you ask questions of your nurse or doctor about your health or health care?					
17. Do you answer questions that are asked by the doctor, nurse, or clinic staff?					
18. Do you ask your doctor or nurse to explain things more clearly if you do not understand their instructions to you?					
19. Do you tell the doctor or nurse whether you followed their advice or recommendations?					
20. Do you explain your health history to your healthcare providers (including past surgeries, allergies, and medications)?					

Please circle how you feel about the following statements

	Not at all important	Not too important	Somewhat important	Important	Very Important
How important is it to you to manage your own health care?	1	2	3	4	5
How confident do you feel about your ability to manage your own health care?	1	2	3	4	5

© Wood, Reiss, & Livingood, McBee, Johnson, 2020

Figure 3.11.2 Transition Readiness Assessment Questionnaire. Reproduced with kind permission from Dr. David L. Wood.

Following are some pointers for transition for the individual with CP:

- Try to get help from your pediatric care team (and possibly others) to connect with the best health professionals to care for you in adulthood.
- You might find it useful to make a summary of your CP and relevant medical history with someone who knows your experience, such as a parent or health professional. When meeting new health professionals, it is helpful to have a short (one- to two-minute) summary of your health care journey to date that can help guide the conversation, or, if easier, a one-page written summary (written by you) to hand to a new health professional. Keep a copy for yourself, and take both copies to the appointment. This summary should include your diagnosis, associated problems, history of treatments, current challenges, and more. This information is very helpful to the new health professional to better help you.
- Find out about the roles of different health professionals and how they might help you.
- Be open and honest and tell the new health professionals everything. You are the expert on your health. The more information you give them the better they can meet your needs.
- If you notice any changes in your condition or any problems such as pain, visit your primary care provider or a PM&R specialist* for advice. Don't wait and see.
- Learning how to advocate for yourself is important in health, just as it is in other parts of your life. Being prepared to advocate for your needs and make decisions about your health can give you more control over your quality of life. To help you advocate, you might practice; for example, you could explain your CP and medical history to someone you trust. Remember to stay calm and polite but assert yourself to get the support or information you need.
- Make a list of all the things you need to keep yourself healthy, such as being physically active, eating well, socializing, taking part in hobbies, working, and resting. By thinking about these, you can start to understand what positively and negatively affects your CP and find a good balance between your condition and lifestyle.

---

* PM&R aims to enhance and restore functional ability and quality of life among those with physical disabilities.

Got Transition is a US federally funded national resource center for health care transition. Its aim is to improve transition from pediatric to adult health care through the use of evidence-driven strategies for health professionals, adolescents, young adults, and their families. The website has a lot of useful guidance.

In its *Lifespan Journal Digest*, the American Academy of Cerebral Palsy and Developmental Medicine routinely spotlight recent studies focused on lifespan issues, including the transition to adult care and aging with a disability.

Links to both these resources are included in **Useful web resources**.

When it comes to the overall management of the person with spastic diplegia, no matter how hard we try, we cannot mitigate the effects of the brain injury. No matter how much we might want to, we cannot "treat and fix" our child. Spastic diplegia cannot (currently) be cured, but with good management its effects can be reduced. As a parent, it is important to be clear on what you can and cannot do to make a difference in your child's life.

Looking back, I wish I'd had a much clearer sense of what we could and could not change and how I, as a parent, could best contribute to Tommy's management and care. Spastic diplegia is very complex, and I am still learning. In retrospect, I see a number of things I would have done differently.

The following are some thoughts on the management of spastic diplegia in childhood and adolescence. They are largely gleaned from my personal experience, particularly of the "make mistakes and learn from them" variety. They are presented in no particular order.

Thinking philosophically

Play to the strengths of your child. Focus on strengths rather than deficits, on what your child can do rather than what they can't do. Focusing on strengths means fostering your child's interests. One of our duties as parents is to help our child discover their passions by allowing them to try different things and then supporting them in what they choose to pursue.

Having a glass-half-full attitude serves us so well in life. With effort, so much is possible. One of my overarching beliefs is that the person with spastic diplegia can largely be anything they want to be. The sky's the limit. I also think the child with spastic diplegia has to be a "despite it" kid—they have to know that despite their spastic diplegia, they will succeed. Indeed, we all need to be "despite it" people in life.

I have always felt that the greatest gift you can give any child is the gift of self-confidence. Your child with spastic diplegia may have a higher hill to climb to achieve it, but you, the parent, can greatly help them on their way.

It is worth keeping in mind that scientific studies generally present the average of outcomes. The gross motor development curves, for example, are based on averages. Be realistic in your goals for your child, but do not limit your aspirations to the average. Aim for the top of the range. It may or may not be possible to get there, but, as with any field of endeavor, the first step toward success is aiming high. Do not let your knowledge of averages limit your child's potential.

You may not see improvement day to day, or even week to week, but when improvement does happen, it is very sweet. These improvements are skills that typically developing children acquire when you're not even looking, and—aside from the big milestone of walking—they are often taken for granted. With Tommy, I stopped taking things for granted and began to notice and appreciate every little change.

We go to great lengths to help our child walk—in other words, to achieve ordinariness. One has to go to extraordinary lengths to achieve ordinariness. Sometimes friends and extended family members may not fully understand.

Resisting the urge to be overprotective

Children learn by making mistakes, as we all do. The typically developing toddler learns to walk while (and by) toppling a lot: they get a sense of their limbs in space, threats to their balance, and how to negotiate obstacles. Because a child with spastic diplegia has difficulty with fluid movement and may have balance issues, we should be careful not to become overprotective and unintentionally stifle their opportunities to learn from movement mistakes. We have to let them fall and learn from falling.

In Tommy's early days at school, he could sense that the staff supervising outdoor play were always very close by. Even as a young child, he sensed they were being overprotective. I asked the school to allow him to play freely, adding that we would not hold them responsible in any way for falls or fractures. It worked. Tommy played much more freely after that, and as it happened, he never did get injured.

Guarding against being overprotective applies throughout life. We need to swing the pendulum the other way and foster independence right from the start. Again, others will take their cues from us. The principle of person-centered care is one we parents must emulate at home: it encourages us to actively involve our child in decision-making related to their care and foster their independence in all areas of life from an early age. Indeed, this principle should apply to all of our children.

Resisting the urge to do too much for the child

I would encourage parents to resist the temptation to do too much for your child. It is much faster, for example, to dress the young child than to allow them to do it themselves. (This was an impulse I very much had to resist.) But it is important the child learn to perform movements and practice the skill, even though the task will take longer. Breaking down dressing tasks and doing each movement correctly, ensuring both hands are involved if one hand is stronger, is an excellent exercise.

We have to develop patience. This applies to parenting across the board, but the temptation to do things for your child is even greater when they have spastic diplegia. Most parents are time-poor, but recognizing the importance of giving your child these opportunities to practice and learn will pay dividends down the line.

In conclusion, the child becomes the adolescent, who in turn becomes the adult. How we look after the child with spastic diplegia will have repercussions long after childhood has ended. Recall the quotation at the beginning of this chapter: the child truly is the father of the man.

Key points Chapter 3

- It is important to understand what best practice in the medical care of individuals with spastic diplegia looks like. Best practice currently includes family-centered care and person-centered care, a multidisciplinary team approach, evidence-based medicine and shared decision-making, data-driven decision-making, specialist centers, early intervention, setting goals, and measurement tools and measuring outcome.
- While a lot of attention is given to development of movement and posture and secondary musculoskeletal problems, for some individuals with spastic diplegia, difficulties with communication or learning may pose bigger barriers to participation.
- Monitoring musculoskeletal development is a constant throughout childhood and adolescence.
- Hip and spine surveillance (monitoring) are important and should start early in life.
- There are two main peaks in the management of the musculoskeletal problems of spastic diplegia. The first occurs in early childhood, when tone reduction (in conjunction with other treatments such as PT and orthoses) is very important. The second occurs in later childhood (at approximately 8 to 12 years), when orthopedic surgery may be needed.
- Orthopedic surgery becomes necessary when the muscle and bone problems (the secondary problems) can no longer be adequately managed by more conservative means, and they are having a significant adverse effect on gait and function.
- Single-event multilevel surgery (SEMLS) involves multiple orthopedic surgical procedures performed during a single operation. Surgeons try to correct all the bone and muscle problems in the same surgical event to avoid multiple hospital admissions, repeated anesthesia, and multiple rehabilitations. SEMLS is now considered best practice for orthopedic surgery in CP.
- SEMLS does not alter the primary problems of CP, and a gradual recurrence of some muscle and bone problems may occur in a proportion of individuals after SEMLS.
- The home program (including exercise and physical activity) is a constant in the life of the child and adolescent with spastic diplegia.

Chapter 4

The adult with spastic diplegia

Introduction

> I don't think motor neurone disease can be an advantage to anyone,
> but it was less of a disadvantage to me than to other people,
> because it did not stop me doing what I wanted.
> **Stephen Hawking**

CP is diagnosed in childhood and is a lifelong condition. It is often thought of as a children's condition, but it is not. People with CP who walk during childhood tend to have a relatively normal life expectancy.[283] If one considers a normal life span to be 80 years, that means for every child and adolescent with CP there are approximately three adults with the condition.

The World Health Organization (WHO) defines an adult as a person older than 19 years of age.[284] But what does being an adult really mean?

While everybody's path in life is different, one description of being an adult includes the following accomplishments:[285]

Completing formal education, entering the labor force, living independently, having romantic relationships and sexual experiences, getting married and having children, establishing peer and family relationships, participating in recreation/leisure, driving a car, and enjoying group social encounters.

Preparing our children to become independent adults is the ultimate goal of most parents—and that's a realistic goal for the parents of the majority of children with spastic diplegia. However, while this chapter focuses on the majority, it is important to remember that a small minority of adults with spastic diplegia have moderate to severe intellectual problems, and therefore they will likely need supported living arrangements, legal guardianship, and support with decision-making.

As a person with spastic diplegia reaches adulthood and skeletal growth has ceased, a certain stabilization of the musculoskeletal aspects of the condition occurs. The rate of change of the condition is slower in adulthood, assuming the adult remains physically active.

People with spastic diplegia may, however, develop secondary conditions in adulthood. Some of these are consistent with typical aging, but some may be unique. Each may influence body systems in more complex ways because of the interactions with CP itself.

The Centers for Disease Control and Prevention (CDC) explain secondary conditions as follows:[286]

As a result of having a specific type of disability, such as a spinal cord injury ... other physical or mental health conditions can occur. Some of these other health conditions are also called secondary conditions ...

The specific secondary conditions that may develop depend on the primary condition. For example, eye problems are secondary conditions that may develop from having diabetes; osteoarthritis (the breakdown of cartilage in the joints) is a secondary condition that may develop from having spastic diplegia.

This chapter addresses the secondary conditions associated with spastic diplegia. Note that the secondary conditions referred to here are general health conditions and separate from the secondary musculoskeletal problems that develop as a result of the primary brain injury in CP, addressed in Chapters 2 and 3.

The development of secondary conditions is not inevitable. Good management can help prevent or minimize their development. Though they are addressed in this chapter on adulthood, some secondary conditions may appear earlier in life.

In childhood and adolescence, growth is the major challenge for the person with spastic diplegia. In adulthood, typical aging becomes the main challenge. Though there are far more adults than children with CP, most of the efforts of health care professionals are directed at children and adolescents.

Meeting the needs of young people with CP is absolutely essential, but given that CP is a lifelong condition and further issues may arise with age, the medical establishment must better address the lack of service provision for adults with CP. To that end, currently, a clinical practice guideline for adults with CP is being developed. Once published, the guideline will, hopefully, pave the way for better service provision for adults with CP.

In addition to the challenge of reduced service provisions, there are significant personal, societal, and economic costs associated with suboptimal health. For example, as addressed in section 4.3, adults with spastic diplegia are underemployed.

If the moral argument for improving service provision and, thus, quality of life for adults with spastic diplegia is not sufficiently persuasive, then perhaps the economic argument will be. Novak and colleagues in 2016 reported that care, loss of income, and tax revenue losses for individuals with CP cost the Australian and American economies $87 billion per year.[287] That cost has likely increased.

Much of the limited research in CP to date has focused on children. An analysis of National Institutes of Health (NIH)* funding for CP research from 2001 to 2013 found that only 4 percent of available funding went toward studies of CP in adulthood.[288] As well, as was noted earlier in

---

* The NIH is the primary US body responsible for health research.

this book, funding generally for CP research is very low relative to the prevalence of the condition and its impact across the life span.

While research on CP in adulthood is considerably less than in childhood, it has been growing over time, as shown by the increase in the annual number of studies from a search using the terms "cerebral palsy" and "adult." See Figure 4.1.1.

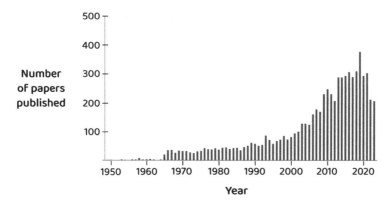

Figure 4.1.1 Number of studies on CP in adulthood per year (PubMed).*

More research is needed to fully understand how CP changes in adulthood and what can be done to prevent or minimize the problems that arise as adults with CP age. Because "adults" range in age from 19 to 80-plus years, they are not a homogenous group. It is necessary to have a better sense of how health care challenges evolve across the decades. Longitudinal research studies for adults with CP as they age would offer valuable information.

A 2008 workshop to define the challenges of treating and preventing secondary conditions in adults with CP concluded with this very worthy goal:[289]

> *The same sense of responsibility and compassion that motivated the research that led to such advances as increasing the survival rates of very low birth weight infants must now be applied to developing the best means of caring for children with CP as they reach adulthood … The medical and research communities have*

---

* A free online database of medical and life sciences research articles.

helped these individuals survive. It is now our responsibility to help them thrive and live productive lives, as uninhibited as possible by the chronic pain and secondary conditions associated with CP.

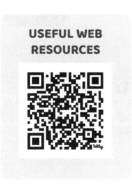

USEFUL WEB RESOURCES

Aging in the typical population

With mirth and laughter let old wrinkles come.
William Shakespeare

The *Oxford English Dictionary* defines aging as "the process of growing old." But that doesn't give us much information. The fact that decline occurs with age is obvious from observing those around us and from seeing how the performance of elite athletes declines relatively early in life. Before addressing aging in adults with CP, let us first look at aging in the typical population.

Examples of the decline that may occur with age include sarcopenia (loss of skeletal muscle mass and strength), joint pain, osteoarthritis, osteoporosis, falls, and low-trauma fractures (easily acquired bone breaks). Many conditions become more prevalent as people age, including cardiovascular disease, cancer, respiratory disease, and diabetes. These conditions are termed "noncommunicable diseases" (NCDs).

Some of the above can be considered part of "normal" aging (e.g., sarcopenia), but most are diagnosable medical conditions. Diagnosable medical conditions occur in the typical population, but they are not "normal." This section addresses sarcopenia, osteoporosis, and NCDs in more detail.

Sarcopenia

Sarcopenia is the loss of skeletal muscle mass and strength.[290] Typically developing adults achieve peak muscle mass by their early 40s, which progressively declines and results in as much as 50 percent loss by the time they are in their 80s. As we saw earlier, muscle strength is related to muscle size. Losing muscle mass has consequences for maintaining the level of function we need to carry out activities of daily living as we age; for example, lifting and carrying objects or even just getting up from a chair. By performing simple muscle strengthening exercises, adults can offset the natural loss of muscle mass that commonly occurs with age.

Protein is required for muscle growth. Older people are less efficient than younger people at extracting protein from food, which means older people need to be especially vigilant about meeting their daily protein needs.[291] For adults over age 65, an average daily intake of at least 1 to 1.2 grams of protein per kilogram of body weight is recommended.*[292]

Osteoporosis

Bone fractures as a result of falls are closely linked to osteoporosis (addressed in sections 2.7 and 3.9). The risk of falling increases with age due to factors such as decreasing muscle strength and balance. Maintaining muscle strength and balance is therefore very important for preventing falls. The consequences of a fall can lead to further complications—for example, a broken leg may lead to much-reduced activity, or a broken wrist may lead to difficulties with self-care. Either may lead to reduced independence. Fear of falling can be another consequence, which may lead to self-imposed restrictions on activity.[293]

---

* For example, a person over 65 weighing 57 kg (126 lb) requires 60 g (just over 2 oz) of protein per day

The AACPDM (American Academy for Cerebral Palsy and Developmental Medicine) has published a care pathway, "Osteoporosis in Cerebral Palsy," and a link to it is included in **Useful web resources.**

Noncommunicable diseases

A noncommunicable disease (NCD) is a medical condition not caused by an infectious agent.* NCDs, also known as chronic diseases, tend to be of long duration. The World Health Organization reported that NCDs are the cause of over three-quarters of all deaths globally. The following four conditions account for over 80 percent of all deaths due to NCDs:[294]

- Cardiovascular disease (e.g., heart attack and stroke)
- Cancer
- Respiratory disease (e.g., chronic obstructive pulmonary disease and asthma)
- Diabetes

In section 1.3, we examined the difference between causes and risk factors. NCDs share four behavioral risk factors:[294]

- Tobacco use
- Physical inactivity
- Unhealthy diet
- Excess alcohol consumption

People have control over each of these risk factors—they are lifestyle choices. However, it is important to acknowledge that socioeconomic factors can adversely affect nutrition and health. Very often, multiple combinations may be present, such as an unhealthy diet combined with physical inactivity.

Cardiometabolic risk factors ("cardio" refers to heart and "metabolic," refers to the process the body uses to turn food into energy) include:

- High levels of blood cholesterol (a type of fat in the blood)

---

* A communicable disease is caused by an infectious agent such as a bacterium or virus.

- High levels of triglycerides (another type of fat in the blood)
- High blood pressure (also termed "hypertension")
- Insulin resistance* or diabetes
- Being overweight or obese†
- Metabolic syndrome (a person is diagnosed with metabolic syndrome if they have at least three of the five risk factors above)
- High levels of C-reactive protein (a protein in the blood; high levels are a sign of inflammation in the body)

In addition to good lifestyle choices, regular health checks with a primary care provider are important for managing our health as we age. A primary care provider will check many of the above risk factors. Most developed countries also have screening programs for many cancers, such as breast and colon cancer. Appropriate health checks and screening can lead to early identification and therefore earlier treatment of conditions.

Finally, not everything goes downhill as we age. Wisdom, sense of self, and comfort in one's own skin generally increase as we get older. Happiness appears to follow a U-shaped trajectory (also known as a "happiness curve"), declining from the optimism of youth to a slump in middle age, then rising again around age 50.[295]

> Generally, we all hope to live a long life, but we also want the quality of those later years to be good. In other words, we want quantity and quality. Whether we like it or not, we all age—but how we age differs. Good lifestyle choices play an important role in preventing many of the health conditions of typical aging described above. Aging is inevitable, but how we age is not—we can choose how we age.

---

* Insulin resistance is the body's reduced responsiveness to insulin, potentially leading to higher than normal blood sugar levels.

† Measured by body mass index (BMI) and/or central obesity. BMI is calculated by dividing a person's body mass in kilograms by the square of their body height in meters. A large waistline (≥ 40 in/102 cm for men and ≥ 35 in/89 cm for women) is a measure of central obesity. This body type is also known as "apple-shaped," as opposed to "pear-shaped," in which fat is deposited on the hips and buttocks. Apple-shaped people are known to be more at risk for cardiometabolic disease than pear-shaped people. A CDC resource on weight is included in **Useful web resources.**

Aging with spastic diplegia

You are never too old to set another goal or to dream a new dream.

C.S. Lewis

Adults with spastic diplegia are not a homogenous group. They range in age from 20 to 80-plus years. They vary in how their condition was managed during childhood and adolescence. They also vary in personality, level of drive, determination, perseverance, and interest in self-care. This is no different from nondisabled adults or those with other primary conditions such as diabetes.

Adults with spastic diplegia have had their condition since childhood, but they are also susceptible to the same challenges of aging as their nondisabled peers. For the person with spastic diplegia, it is almost as if, on entering adulthood, two roads converge: the challenges of growing up with the condition meet the challenges of typical aging. The adult with spastic diplegia must manage these two sets of challenges in combination. The problems of aging may occur at a younger age and with more severity in adults with CP than in those without the condition.[296] A recent systematic review and meta-analysis* of 69 studies from 18 countries found that the prevalence of several chronic physical and mental health conditions was higher among adults with CP than those without CP.[297] However, much can be done to prevent or minimize many of the secondary conditions that can arise.

The management and treatment of spastic diplegia in childhood and adolescence has improved in recent decades. This influences how today's children and adolescents will fare as tomorrow's adults. The general public's awareness of many health issues has also improved. For example, people today are much more aware of the downsides of smoking and the important contribution of physical exercise to overall health. As in childhood and adolescence, spastic diplegia in adulthood affects not only the individual with the condition but also their family and those in their immediate circle.

On a philosophical note, don't be discouraged when you read statements like, "Nearly one-third of adults with CP had X." Remember, this means more than two-thirds of adults with CP did not have X. That's just as significant. The research tends to focus on the negatives, so it's up to the reader to recognize the unstated positive findings.

If we were to look at the body mass index (BMI) of a group of adults, we would see a normal distribution: a few people might be classed as underweight, some would be normal weight, some overweight, and some obese. The fact that many people are not at the ideal weight does not mean you cannot be. Similarly, as you read about the results of studies in this chapter, please use them to inform but not limit you.

This section addresses the following challenges of aging with spastic diplegia:

- **Musculoskeletal decline**
- **Mobility**

---

* A systematic review summarizes the results of several scientific studies on the same topic. It can be qualitative (descriptive) or quantitative (numerical). The quantitative approach is called a meta-analysis.

- Falls
- Pain
- Noncommunicable diseases and risk factors
- Fatigue
- Depression and anxiety
- Quality of life and health-related quality of life
- Participation
- Areas of unmet need

Though these challenges will be addressed separately, they are very much interdependent.

Musculoskeletal decline

Chapter 2 addressed the primary, secondary, and tertiary problems of spastic diplegia. Chapter 3 addressed the optimal management of the condition in childhood and adolescence. The aim is to arrive at adulthood (when bone growth ceases) with the best possible musculoskeletal alignment. If correction of the muscle and bone deformities is not addressed (or not fully addressed) during childhood and adolescence, they may persist into adulthood.[298] These muscle and bone problems may cause further decline in mobility as well as pain, fatigue, and other problems in adulthood. As people age, further coping responses (tertiary problems) may develop to compensate for decreased muscle strength and deterioration in balance. However, as we will see in the next section, orthopedic surgery to address muscle and bone problems is still possible in adulthood.

The conditions that occur in typically aging adults can have even greater implications for adults with spastic diplegia. For example:

- **Sarcopenia** (loss of skeletal muscle mass and strength): For individuals with spastic diplegia, muscle mass and strength have been challenges since childhood. In adulthood, these individuals acquire the added challenge of loss of muscle mass and strength due to aging. Hip and knee extension strength was found to be considerably lower (less than 75 percent of normal) among adolescents and young adults with spastic CP.[299] Maximum plantar flexor strength was found to be approximately 50 percent less in young adults with spastic CP (average age 25) than in typically developing young adults, and approximately 35 percent less than in typically developing adults above age 70.[300]

- **Osteoarthritis:** The prevalence of osteoarthritis among middle-age adults with CP (GMFCS levels I to III) was 33 percent.[301] In another study, the age-adjusted prevalence of arthritis was found to be significantly greater among adults with CP than among those without CP: 31 percent versus 17 percent.[302]

- **Osteoporosis or osteopenia:** The prevalence of osteoporosis or osteopenia among middle-age adults with CP GMFCS levels I to III was 32 percent.[301] Adults with CP had a higher incidence of osteoporosis compared with adults without CP.[303]

- **Fractures** Adults with CP (no breakdown by type) had a higher prevalence of fractures compared with adults without CP: 6 percent versus 3 percent.[304]

Mobility

Retaining the ability to walk (independently or using mobility aids) for at least household distances is important for independence. A systematic review and meta-analysis found that 56 percent of adults with CP experienced a perceived decline in walking over time.[305] Those with worse initial gait ability, bilateral (rather than unilateral) motor impairment, older age, and higher levels of pain or fatigue were at higher risk of gait decline.[306] The decline occurred earlier in adults with CP than in typically aging peers.[306]

Self-reported factors perceived as causes of decline in walking in adulthood included balance problems, pain, increased spasticity, decline in muscle strength, contractures or joint deformity, stiffness, fatigue, knee problems, fractures due to falls, fear of falling or falls, and reduced fitness and endurance.[306] The reasons for decline in walking in adulthood may differ from those in adolescence. (We examined reasons for decline in walking in adolescence in section 2.9, including the unfavorable strength-to-mass ratio that develops as the child grows.)

People who engage in regular physical activity were found to be at lower risk of experiencing decline in mobility. Deterioration in gait was strongly associated with inactivity.[306] In other words, mobility and physical activity are intricately linked. Thorpe reported that a disabling condition such as CP frequently causes a "cycle of deconditioning" (loss of fitness) in which physical function deteriorates, followed by a further decrease in physical activity and a cascade of increasing functional decline.[307] All of the above emphasizes how critical it is to remain physically active throughout adulthood.

Elsewhere it has been noted that individuals at GMFCS levels I and II are at lower risk of gait deterioration and generally continue to walk in their 60s.[308] Loss of walking skills in the adult with CP appears to occur at two peaks.[308] The first, at around age 20 to 25, is commonly associated with progressive crouch gait and an inability to keep up with one's peers in the community, workplace, and academic settings. The second peak, around age 40 to 45, is commonly associated with progressive fatigue, pain, and possibly accelerated joint degeneration, which prevents further functional walking.

Preserving mobility in adulthood might require the use of mobility aids the person may not have needed before.

Falls

Earlier we saw that balance is affected in spastic diplegia. Although adults with CP may have become somewhat used to falling (and are more aware of situations where they are at risk of falling and how to protect themselves when falling), it tends to be more socially uncomfortable when a fall occurs. In addition, for reasons of physics, an adult is more likely to be injured from a fall than a child. Citing from a number of studies on falls:

- Fifty-six percent of adults with spastic bilateral CP had fallen at least once in the past month and 81 percent had fallen more than five times in the past year.[309]
- Adults with CP are four times more likely to fall, and they fall more often, than adults without CP.[310]
- Fall frequency in ambulatory adults with CP was two to threefold higher than in adults without CP (GMFCS levels I to III, 29 percent spastic diplegia).[311]

Falls occur naturally with aging, but they usually occur later in life in adults who do not have a disability and who have better overall health and fitness. The incidence of falls is higher for people with CP at younger ages[310,312] and may be more common if they do not use mobility aids.

Psychological effects of falls include embarrassment and loss of confidence.[311] Additionally, the fear of falling is a real concern in adulthood when responsibilities and activities change. For example, when pregnant and/or caring for an infant, the fear of falling is great due to the increased consequences.

Falling continues to be a challenge for Tommy. Thankfully, he is aware of the risks and takes precautions—he is particularly careful around stairs or traffic. Tommy had one bad fall, where he fell backward and hit his head against a glass coffee table, which broke on impact. The resulting cut required stapling at the local emergency room.

Pain

A systematic review and meta-analysis reported a pain prevalence of 65 percent among adults with CP, though studies report different prevalence depending on their definition of pain.[305] Studies report higher levels of pain among adults with CP compared with the general population: 28 percent versus 15 percent;[313] 75 percent versus 39 percent;[314] and 44 percent versus 28 percent.[302] Adults with diplegia reported pain in the back (64 percent), neck (38 percent), foot/ankle (54 percent), shoulder (38 percent), knee (41 percent), hip (35 percent), arm (22 percent), head (25 percent), and other (6 percent).[313]

Pain is a major determinant of quality of life and affects physical and mental functioning. It leads to reduced productivity and concentration.[285] Pain may lead to problems with sleep, which causes fatigue, which can further exacerbate pain.

Pain negatively impacts activity, mental health, and employment in adults with CP.[315,316,317] CP alone does not predict reduced quality of life. However, adults with CP who have pain have reduced quality of life, and increased prevalence of pain with age coincides with decline in quality of life from childhood to adulthood.[318,319]

Noncommunicable diseases and risk factors

Recall that noncommunicable diseases (NCDs) are medical conditions that are not caused by infectious agents, and they are generally chronic. A systematic review and meta-analysis reported the prevalence of several chronic conditions among ambulatory adults with CP: obesity (20 percent), hypercholesterolemia (high cholesterol, 26 percent), and hypertension (high blood pressure, 10 percent).[297]

A study by Cremer and colleagues of adults in the US with CP GMFCS levels I to III (demographic details in Table 4.3.1) reported chronic condition prevalence by gender as shown in Figure 4.3.1.[301] The prevalence of chronic conditions was higher among women than men for five of the seven conditions. It is worth noting that prevalence rates may vary by country.

Table 4.3.1 Demographics of adults in the Cremer study

	WOMEN	MEN
Number of participants	112	94
Average age (years)	50	48
Body mass index (BMI) kg/m²	31	27
% obese (BMI>30)	44	18
% smokers	14	16

Data from Cremer and colleagues.[301]

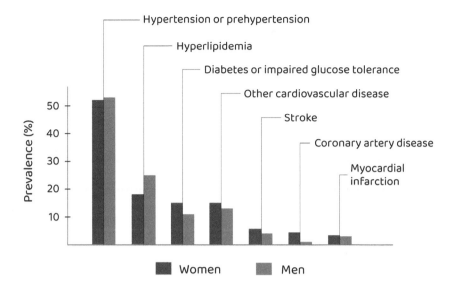

Figure 4.3.1 Prevalence (percent) of chronic conditions in adults with CP GMFCS levels I to III, by gender. Data from Cremer and colleagues.[301] **Hypertension** is a condition characterized by high blood pressure. **Prehypertension** is a condition characterized by blood pressure levels that are elevated but not yet classified as hypertension. **Hyperlipidemia** is a condition characterized by high levels of fats in the blood. **Impaired glucose tolerance** refers to a prediabetes condition where blood sugars are higher than normal but not high enough for a diabetes diagnosis. **Myocardial infarction** is also known as heart attack.

Multimorbidity is defined as the presence of two or more chronic conditions.[297] The prevalence of multimorbidity was significantly higher among obese than nonobese adults with CP GMFCS levels I to III (76 percent versus 54 percent).[301]

Using data from 2002 to 2010, Peterson and colleagues reported the age-adjusted prevalence of eight chronic conditions among adults in the US with and without CP.[302] (See Figure 4.3.2.) The prevalence of the eight chronic conditions was higher among adults with CP. It's understandable why adults with CP might have a higher burden of joint pain and arthritis, but the remaining conditions do not have a direct link to the condition. However, as we will see, lower levels of activity due to CP lead to lower fitness. Since people who are less active and less fit have a higher incidence of diabetes, hypertension, and cardiovascular disease, it makes sense that CP puts people at increased risk of these conditions.

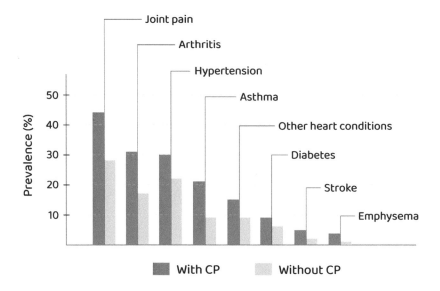

Figure 4.3.2 Age-adjusted prevalence of chronic conditions in adults with and without CP. Data from Peterson and colleagues.[302] **Age-adjusted** refers to a data standardization method to account for differences in ages allowing for more accurate comparison. **Emphysema** is a condition in which the air sacs of the lungs are damaged and enlarged, causing breathlessness.

There is ample evidence to suggest that the burden of NCDs and their risk factors are higher among ambulatory adults with CP compared with the general population.[297]

Fatigue

Fatigue describes feeling exhausted, tired, weak, or lacking energy.[320] A study found that adults with CP had significantly more physical fatigue, but not more mental fatigue, than the general population.[320] Additionally, adults with a moderate grade of CP had a higher prevalence of fatigue than adults with mild or severe CP, suggesting that those with moderate CP may try to minimize their disability to keep up with their peers.[320] Crouch gait has been associated with high fatigue in adults with spastic diplegia.[321] One study emphasized the importance of physical activity and good weight management to both prevent and treat fatigue in adults with CP.[322] This was consistent with the findings of earlier fatigue studies.[167,320,323]

Depression and anxiety

Depression is a common and serious mood disorder. It can affect how a person feels and thinks, and it influences activities such as sleeping, eating, and working.[324] For a depression diagnosis, the symptoms must be present for at least two weeks.[324] Adults with spastic bilateral CP in the Netherlands were found to have a higher prevalence of depressive symptoms than the general population (25 percent versus 12 percent).[314] A UK study found that only adults with CP and without intellectual disability have a higher risk of developing depression than adults who do not have CP.[325] However, a US study found no such difference between adults with CP and the general population (where the rate of depression in both groups was 20 percent).[326]

Occasional anxiety is normal; however, anxiety disorders are more than just occasional worry or fear. There are several types of anxiety disorders, each with distinct symptoms and triggers.[327] The same UK study found that only adults with CP and without intellectual disability were found to have a higher risk of developing anxiety than adults who do not have CP.[325]

Quality of life and health-related quality of life

Quality of life and health-related quality of life are two different concepts.

Quality of life (QOL) is defined as "the individual's perception of their position in life in the context of the culture and value system in which they live, and in relation to their goals, expectations, standards, and concerns."[157] Very little research has been conducted on QOL in adults with CP,[8,328] and the research that does exist does not paint a clear picture. Reduced QOL has been reported among adults with bilateral CP compared with the general population.[321]

Health-related quality of life (HRQOL) is defined as "the way in which a condition (almost always a chronic condition) affects a person's well-being."[8] A person may have reduced HRQOL because of the impact a condition has on their physical and/or mental functioning, but they may still have a high QOL because they are perfectly happy with their life. In other words, there are factors beyond health that make up a person's perception of their QOL. A study showed low perceived HRQOL for physical functioning but not mental functioning among adults with bilateral CP.[329] Higher general self-efficacy (a greater willingness to expend effort to achieve behavior) was related to higher physical and mental HRQOL.

Participation

Participation is one of the three levels of human functioning identified in the ICF (addressed in section 1.8). Participation restrictions are problems an individual may experience in their involvement in life situations. Employment, relationships, and having children are indicators of participation in society.

A Dutch study of individuals with CP without intellectual disability found that individuals at GMFCS levels I and II achieved autonomy in adulthood in most participation domains (leisure, transportation, finances, education and employment, housing, and intimate relationships). However, with regard to intimate relationships, they had slightly less experience (approximately 80 percent of individuals) than age-matched peers (approximately 90 percent).[330] A Swedish study of 1,888 adults with CP, age 16 to 78, however, reported different results for participation.[331] See Table 4.3.2.

Table 4.3.2 Participation for adults with CP GMFCS levels I to III

AREA OF LIFE	GMFCS LEVEL I (%)	GMFCS LEVEL II (%)	GMFCS LEVEL III (%)
Having no partner	77	82	84
Housing			
Independent	40	41	47
With parents	51	39	34
Assisted living	7	18	15
Other	2	3	4
Personal assistance			
None	98	80	54
>160 hours per week	1	6	11
Occupation			
Mainstream education	39	18	15
Special education	5	9	10
Competitive employment	27	18	17
Supported employment	4	3	3
Activity center	14	39	34
No occupation	11	14	21
For all the above, the proportion full time	71	52	52

Data from Pettersson and Rodby-Bousquet.[331]

While there are no comparable figures for the typical population, the levels of participation can be assumed to be lower. For example, a high percentage of those with CP GMFCS levels I to III, did not have a partner, and this applied across all age groups.

Employment is important for many reasons, including financial independence, social interaction, self-esteem, and sense of self, but it may also have implications for future health care and retirement costs. Very often, the barriers to employment are small and require only simple accommodations—a high percentage (59 percent) of accommodations cost absolutely nothing to make while the rest typically cost only $500 per employee.[332] Indeed, research shows that companies that embrace employees with disabilities clearly see the results in their bottom line. They have higher productivity levels and lower staff turnover rates, are twice as likely to outperform their peers in shareholder returns, and create larger returns on investment.[332]

A Dutch study found that 11 percent of adults with bilateral spastic CP had children compared with approximately 50 percent of the general population.[329] A US study found that women with CP who were surveyed about their desire to have children (30 percent) or had experienced pregnancy (20 percent) exhibited significantly higher functional levels, including mobility, manual dexterity, and communication ability.[333] A higher rate of cesarean section (50 percent), preterm births (12 percent), low birth weight infants (16 percent), and very low birth weight infants (7 percent) were reported by women with CP compared with national statistics.[333] The authors concluded that in addition to the need to discuss and support the desire of women with CP to have sexual relationships and experience pregnancy, there is a need to investigate preterm and low birth weight infants born to women with CP.

Finally, higher general self-efficacy was found to be related to better participation.[329]

Clearly, participation in society is very important and more research is needed, particularly in the area of participation restrictions.

Areas of unmet need

The greatest area of unmet need reported by young adults with CP was information about their condition* (79 percent), followed by mobility (66 percent) and health care (66 percent).[334] The authors suggested that while parents may receive information, they might not be communicating it adequately to their children, leaving them with unanswered questions. Furthermore, a person's questions about CP might change over

---

* For example: complications, consequences, causes of CP.

time as their needs change during adolescence and adulthood. Other studies have reported a similar lack of information during the transition to adulthood,[335,336] underscoring the need for a book like this one, as well as more research on adults with CP.

———

Finally, while the most recent definition of CP is very useful, it may not sufficiently alert us to the secondary conditions that may arise in adulthood. As O'Brien and colleagues explained, the definition was developed to be used in childhood—it was not intended to imply that progressive problems might not appear in adult life.[337]

Management and treatment of spastic diplegia in adulthood

The way we are living, timorous or bold, will have been our life.
Seamus Heaney

This section addresses the management and treatment of spastic diplegia in adulthood, specifically:

- Health services for adults with CP
- Treatments
- The home program
- General pointers

Health services for adults with CP

The general consensus in the literature is that services for adults with CP are extremely limited. Multidisciplinary care teams in place for children and adolescents with CP largely do not exist for adults at a time when their needs are becoming ever more complex. This disparity has been observed in many countries, including Norway,[167] the US,[285] the Netherlands,[338] Ireland,[339] Germany,[340] and Canada.[341] Scandinavian countries are known for their well-developed social health systems, yet other than Sweden,[331] they too experience this fall-off in services. It is very unfortunate that care for people with CP becomes fragmented just as they enter adulthood.

In their 2009 report following a workshop to define the challenges of treating and preventing secondary complications in adults with CP, Tosi and colleagues noted that pediatric facilities are starting to extend their mandate to include adults.[289] They cited Gillette's model of life-time care.[*] Gillette provides lifelong specialty care to adolescents and adults who have conditions that began in childhood. This specialization means that even though Gillette is a lifetime care provider, it does not treat lifelong conditions that develop after early childhood.

For the adult with CP, three different components of health need monitoring:[342]

- Acute health problems (e.g., infections)
- Lifestyle health risks
- Secondary conditions

As has been shown, there is strong evidence that adults with spastic diplegia encounter more and earlier health problems than their typically aging peers, and these problems affect a broad range of areas spanning all ICF levels. But much can still be done to prevent, minimize, or deal with these challenges. However, because of limited specialist health services for adults with CP, they must take great personal responsibility for their own health and well-being.

It has been reported in the literature that health care professionals often blame their CP diagnosis for just about all the symptoms and problems that develop in adulthood.[343,344] Rosenbaum noted: "We hear too many stories from adults with cerebral palsy whose abdominal pain, for example, was assumed to be 'part of (your) cerebral palsy,' when in fact they had treatable Crohn's or gall bladder disease."[344] It is important to

---

* The Gillette adult clinic is a lifelong outpatient clinic for those age 16 and older who have conditions that began in childhood. It includes access to an inpatient unit for adults age 18 to 40. Specialists may provide care to adults whom they previously treated as children.

ensure that the cause of a health problem is not wrongly attributed to CP when there may be another cause.

Sometimes, changes with aging versus new neurological changes are difficult to separate, especially in adults with CP who are older than 40 years, but it is important to determine the cause.[345] New neurological changes might include a decreased level of alertness or cognitive functioning, decreased ability to communicate, weakness, or numbness, including paresthesia (pins-and-needles sensation.) For example, cervical myelopathy should be considered with new neurological changes. Cervical myelopathy refers to the symptoms related to spinal cord compression (myelopathy) in the neck (cervical) region. Symptoms may include weakness, numbness, loss of fine motor skills, and bladder issues. In addition, dual diagnoses (for example, multiple sclerosis* or even genetic conditions) should also be considered with functional decline.[345]

All adults—those with and without disabilities—should attend regular health screenings (e.g., for cancers, bone health, and sexually transmitted infections) and have an annual medical checkup with their primary care provider. Research has found that many adults with CP do not receive adequate health checks and screening.[289,346,347]

Addressing medical caregivers, Murphy succinctly summarized the situation: "It should be a humbling revelation to all caregivers that this population of adults is almost certainly under-studied, under-screened, and under-diagnosed."[343] (Note that "underdiagnosis" here refers to other conditions, not CP.)

Because of their higher risk of osteoporosis, people with spastic diplegia need to be attentive to bone health. It is recommended that adults with CP have at least an annual bone health assessment (including medical history, lifestyle review, nutrition, and, as needed, evaluation for any concerning changes in bone health, such as new fractures or medications that affect bone health) with appropriate blood testing and imaging. DXA scans† may be used for surveillance every three to

---

* A chronic autoimmune disease of the central nervous system where the immune system mistakenly attacks the myelin, the protective covering of axons, leading to interruption in the transmission of nerve impulses. See Figure 1.2.2.

† A test that measures bone mineral density.

five years.[348] Good nutrition, ensuring no deficiencies in calcium and vitamin D, and physical activity, especially weight-bearing or impact activities, can help promote good bone health.[271]

Despite these concerns, this optimistic opinion is heartening: "Much improvement in specialty health care for adults with CP has occurred over the past three decades. Surely the best is yet to come."[343]

Treatments

The goals of treatment or intervention for adults with CP are inclusion and participation in major life areas.[285] Objectives include minimizing problems with body functions and structure, preventing secondary conditions, and optimizing activities and participation.

The different treatments for spastic diplegia are reviewed in Chapter 3. Here, we focus on what these treatments look like in adulthood. When planning any treatment, it is important to set SMART goals, as discussed in section 3.2. Note that the goal for a particular treatment may be different in adulthood than in childhood.

a) Physical therapy and occupational therapy

Physical therapy (PT) and occupational therapy (OT) remain very relevant in adulthood and are usually delivered as an episode of care (EOC).[*] Rosenbaum and colleagues described the focus of therapy for adults with CP as helping individuals in areas including employment, relationships, and childbearing. They added that adults with CP may require specific focused surveillance and intervention for pain, joint wear and tear, and general mobility in addition to fitness and recreational activities.[163]

In adulthood, the focus of therapy shifts to guidance and education more than intervention, but both are used as required. Therapists at the Gillette adult clinic provided the following examples of EOCs for adults with CP. In these examples the therapist is acting as an educator in prevention and giving guidance rather than providing intervention.

---

[*] A period of therapy (at the appropriate frequency) followed by a therapy break.

- Instruction in balance, gait, strength-training exercises, and the home program.
- Fall assessment to determine the reasons for falls and offer instruction in balance and strengthening exercises for fall prevention. They can also offer guidance on appropriate mobility aids or orthoses and footwear to prevent falls.
- Pain education and instruction in ways to decrease pain: certain therapists have advanced training in pain management. Many research studies show pain education can greatly decrease chronic pain.[349,350]
- Advice on gentle postural exercises and possible affordable adaptations (e.g., changing the angle of a keyboard or the height of chair or desk for optimal posture).
- Instruction in preservation and strengthening exercises to help prevent overuse injuries; for example, when using a manual wheelchair. (Power-assist wheelchairs can also help prevent overuse injuries.)
- Recommendations for home and environmental adaptations (such as adding handrails, removing throw rugs, or improving lighting).
- Mobility assessment and training on ways to continue to be as independent as possible throughout the day in the home, at work, and in the community.
- Equipment provision; for example, a walker or other gait aid to maintain safe walking and prevent falls, a manual or power-assist wheelchair for long distances, or bathroom equipment for safe showering.
- Driving assessment: driving specialists can assess driving ability, including determining if behind-the-wheel and car adaptations are needed to allow independent driving.

The following are useful pointers on mobility:[351]

- Mobility aids are "tools," and people might benefit from having a variety of options available. For example, an individual may use a walker or wheelchair occasionally for longer distances, in certain environments, or when feeling fatigued. They may choose to use a mobility aid in a way that suits their needs; the decision to use one does not have to be "all or nothing." Part-time use may help with participation.
- A crutch is not a "crutch"—mobility aids are tools that can help the person participate more in everyday life.

- Deciding to use a mobility aid can be a positive rather than a negative step, allowing for greater participation and less pain and fatigue. A wheelchair or motorized scooter can help a person with CP conserve energy, which they can then use to engage with peers or become more involved at school or at work. O'Brien and colleagues noted that:[337]

  [The] decision to become a regular wheelchair user is often a positive step, not a negative one. People in this situation typically report not only reductions in pain and fatigue, but also associated improvements in initiative and self-esteem, consequent upon a decision to elect to use a wheelchair, rather than to struggle on painfully and awkwardly, trying to walk.

- A mobility aid can help prevent falls, excessive sway through the trunk, or overreliance on one limb at the expense of the other. It may help lessen age-related musculoskeletal changes and pain over time.
- Those for whom walking demands a lot of extra energy may sometimes lie awake at night imagining where they will have to walk the next day, expending mental energy as well as physical energy on walking.
- The design of mobility aids has improved over time. Wheelchair design and function, for example, has greatly improved in recent years: modern wheelchairs are smaller, faster, and better designed. There are also sports wheelchairs available.
- Mobility aids can include the use of balance dogs (or service dogs), which are dogs trained to wear a particular harness or handle. The dog and harness can serve as a gait aid or for other tasks as needed. These dogs also know how to brace their backs so that if the person falls or is on the floor they can push off the dog to stand up. There's a lot of work involved in caring for a dog, but they can also serve as an emotional support animal and are often perceived as more socially acceptable than a gait aid. Dogs are also great icebreakers for getting to know other people. A video about a student and her balance dog is included in **Useful web resources**.

b) Tone reduction

Tone reduction may include oral medications, botulinum neurotoxin A (BoNT-A) injection, phenol injection, intrathecal baclofen (ITB), and selective dorsal rhizotomy (SDR). BoNT-A has been shown to be effective in improving spasticity among adults with CP, but there have been mixed results for other functional outcomes.[352]

SDR has been carried out more frequently in children than in adolescents or adults. A study of 21 adults with spastic diplegia who underwent SDR in adulthood concluded that it can be an effective treatment for adults with spastic diplegia who are unresponsive to medical therapy and should be considered as an option in carefully selected patients. Though the study represented the largest series of adult patients with spastic diplegia treated with SDR to date, the authors noted that the data needed to be validated in a larger study.[353] Rehabilitation after SDR progresses more slowly in adulthood than in childhood; this is discussed in more detail below under "Orthopedic surgery."

c) Orthopedic surgery

Adults may have orthopedic surgery to address individual or multiple musculoskeletal problems. Multilevel surgery may be performed on adults. While bilateral (two-sided) surgery is generally carried out in a single operation in children, in adolescents and adults it may be performed sequentially, one side at a time.[259] On the one hand, this approach facilitates rehabilitation as it allows the person to bear weight on one side, allowing them to be more functional after surgery. However, anecdotally, the rehabilitation from the first side surgery may be adversely affected by the remaining musculoskeletal deformities on the other side. Therefore, where possible, bilateral surgery is preferable. Orthopedic surgery to address degenerative joint disease with possible joint replacement can be performed as an isolated procedure or as part of multilevel surgery.

Rehabilitation after surgery (of any type) is more prolonged in adults than in children because adults heal more slowly and their lives are generally more independent with more responsibilities. Children are already dependent on their parents: after SEMLS, they return home to an environment where their needs are already being met by others. This isn't the case for the adult. Since rehabilitation takes considerable time, once the initial rehabilitation is over, the adult may be trying to juggle further rehabilitation with work, caring for family, and other responsibilities.

Significant challenges for independent adults following multilevel surgery include loss of independence, loss of ability to care for others (such as children or elderly parents), and loss of income. Can the adult even "go home"? If going home is not an option (because, for example, there is no one to care for them), where do they go? They can't go to a rehab facility right away because they are non-weight-bearing. A nursing home is often the answer, but this is far from ideal because the adult generally has little in common with typical nursing home residents. Transitional care units (or short-term care facilities) are an option: these are typically set up for people whose medical needs are too intense for home but not intense enough for an acute hospital setting.

Thomason and Graham reported that rehabilitation after multilevel surgery can be an "order of magnitude" more difficult for adolescents and adults than it is for younger children, and that adolescents and adults are more prone to anxiety, depression, and functional regression.[259]

In addition to the age-dependent difference in rehabilitation time, rehabilitation for the same procedure (e.g., knee replacement surgery) can take longer for adults with CP than for their nondisabled peers. This is important to note because adults with CP may expect a rehabilitation period similar to that of their nondisabled peers.

As for outcome, multilevel surgery was found to be an effective and safe procedure to improve gait in adults with bilateral spastic CP and in those who had undergone previous SEMLS in childhood.[340] (The study analyzed short-term outcomes at two years.) Total hip replacement was found to be safe and effective in selected individuals with CP with severe degenerative arthritis.[308] Long-term follow-up studies have shown pain relief of more than 90 percent and improved function with time even in adults as young as 30. Wear and tear to the replacement hip joint was found to be minimal.[308]

Because research funding is limited, very few outcome studies on adults with CP exist. Medical professionals treating adults with CP must rely more on their clinical skill and experience rather than the results of research studies.

The home program

This section needs to be read in conjunction with section 3.5, which details the home program for the adolescent with CP. That information applies equally to the adult with CP. The following are some points specific to adults.

During childhood and adolescence, prolonged stretching is needed to achieve the daily hours of stretch required to keep muscle growth at pace with bone growth until bone growth ceases at around age 20. In adulthood, stretching is recommended for the same reasons as for non-disabled adults: to keep muscles flexible, maintain joint range of motion (ROM), and avoid injury. Even nondisabled people do not fully stretch out their muscles while going about their normal daily lives. A study of adults with CP found that decreased hip flexion ROM may contribute to an increased risk for low back pain.[326] Stretching exercises two to three times per week are recommended for both nondisabled people and those with CP.

The WHO notes that "participation in regular physical activity reduces the risk of coronary heart disease and stroke, diabetes, hypertension, colon cancer, breast cancer, and depression. Additionally, physical activity is a key determinant of energy expenditure and thus is funda-mental to energy balance and weight control."[214] Consistently strong evidence demonstrates that people with CP participate in less physical activity and spend more time engaged in sedentary behavior than their nondisabled peers throughout the life span.[347] Studies have shown that:

- Adults with CP who reported preserved mobility throughout adult-hood attribute it to regular physical activity, participation, and maintenance of strength, balance, and overall fitness.[354]
- Adults with CP who engaged in regular physical activity were at lower risk of decline in mobility. Deterioration in gait was strongly associated with inactivity.[306]

Details of the exercise and physical activity requirements for people with CP, as recommended by Verschuren and colleagues, are included in Table 3.5.2 and are summarized below.[213] The first four requirements are the same as in childhood and adolescence; the fifth is an addition to the list for adults:

- Cardiorespiratory (aerobic) exercise
- Resistance (muscle strengthening) exercise
- Daily moderate to vigorous physical activity
- Avoiding sedentary behavior
- Neuromotor exercise (training balance, agility, and coordination)

The last, neuromotor exercise, is important for all adults, not just those with CP.[214,355] It is particularly important for avoiding falls, which we know can be a problem for adults with CP. A therapist can recommend suitable neuromotor exercises.

General pointers

These pointers assume autonomy is possible, but it is recognized that this is not always the case.

- Try to understand your condition as much as possible, as well as the possible changes that may occur with aging. In a sense, forewarned is forearmed.
- Because services for adults with CP are, unfortunately, extremely limited, you are encouraged to build your own team. Do not wait for services for adults with CP to improve. As noted in Chapter 3, it is important to recognize that you, the person with the condition, are the most vital member of your team. You are responsible for putting your own care team in place. Find and connect with a center that provides services to adults with CP. There may not be one in your area, but take the time to research the best options available. An adult physical medicine and rehabilitation (PM&R) specialist will be able to help you prevent problems and deal with those that may arise. Try to find a good local primary care provider or general practitioner who understands CP for routine general health checks. Find a physical therapist and/or occupational therapist (again, preferably one who has experience working with people with CP) who will be able to support you if, and when, you need it.
- Get a copy of the clinical practice guideline for adults with CP when it becomes available. (It will be available online through the Cerebral Palsy Foundation.)
- Completing and maintaining an exercise and physical activity program is a crucial aspect of self-care. It is something each person

must do for themselves. The benefits of exercise and physical activity accrue at so many levels, from preserving function to cardiometabolic health to preventing secondary conditions. Think of exercise and physical activity as a powerful medication that is available for free. (How many more people would "take" it if they thought of it this way?) The concept of "exercise is medicine" has been recognized since ancient times.

- Getting adequate rest is important. Walking is more demanding for an adult with CP than for a nondisabled adult. Additionally, the amount of exercise and physical activity required demands a lot of energy. It's important to achieve the right balance between activity and rest.

- A healthy diet is important for all adults—nondisabled and those with a disability. This includes adequate hydration. Get dietary advice from a specialist if you need it. Excess weight is not good for anyone, but it is especially taxing for a person with CP. Weight management is important not only for reducing the risk of NCDs but also for better musculoskeletal health and to help maintain walking. Because of their smaller and weaker muscles, people with CP cannot afford to be carrying excess weight. Keeping track of your BMI and central obesity is important. Try to keep your BMI in the healthy range and your waist circumference within recommended limits; all you need is a weighing scale and a measuring tape. It is worth monitoring both metrics because some people with a "normal" BMI can still have an unhealthy level of body fat. Finally, regarding diet, keep in mind that older adults require more protein. Read food labels and be mindful of the amount of protein in what you're eating. It can take some effort to achieve the recommended protein intake.

- Prevent, prevent, prevent. Think of aging with CP like taking care of your teeth. Brushing and flossing every day and visiting the dentist or hygienist regularly are the best ways to prevent tooth decay, but problems may still arise, and when they do, a dentist can help address them. The outcome may not be perfect, but problems can be dealt with. Take the same approach to the management of aging with CP. Be aware of the problems that may arise and work hard to prevent or minimize them. Time spent preventing problems is generally much more effective than time spent dealing with problems. However, if problems do arise, medical professionals can help.

- We each "own" our health. We may be able to get people to clean our house, pack for a move, walk our pets, and perform many more of life's chores, but we cannot get people to do our walking, cycling, or swimming for us. We must own our fitness, BMI, and cardiovascular health. We can call in experts to help, and they may provide valuable guidance, but they do not own our health.
- All adults should strive to maintain participation in society as they age. Try to add friends as you age; our peer groups tend to diminish later in life.
- Finally, as C.S. Lewis put it, remember: "You are never too old to set another goal or to dream a new dream."

Key points Chapter 4

- CP is diagnosed in infancy and is a lifelong condition. It is often thought of as a children's condition, but it is not. If one considers a normal life span, for every child and adolescent with CP there are approximately three adults with the condition.

- As a person with spastic diplegia reaches adulthood and skeletal growth has ceased, a certain stabilization of the musculoskeletal aspects of the condition occurs. The rate of change of the condition is slower in adulthood, assuming the adult remains physically active. People with spastic diplegia may, however, develop secondary conditions in adulthood. Some are consistent with typical aging, some may be unique. Each may influence body systems in more complex ways because of the interactions with CP itself.

- Examples of the decline that may occur with typical aging include sarcopenia, joint pain, osteoarthritis, osteoporosis, falls, and low-trauma fractures. Many conditions become more prevalent as people age, including cardiovascular disease, cancer, respiratory disease, and diabetes. These conditions are termed "noncommunicable diseases."

- Adults with spastic diplegia have had their condition since childhood, but they are also susceptible to the same challenges of typical aging. For the person with spastic diplegia, it is almost as if, on entering adulthood, two roads converge: the challenges of growing up with the condition meet the challenges of typical aging. The adult with spastic diplegia must manage these two sets of challenges in combination. The problems of aging may occur at a younger age and with more severity in adults with CP than in those without the condition.

- The prevalence of several chronic physical and mental health conditions has been found to be higher among adults with CP than those without CP. However, much can be done to prevent or minimize many of the secondary conditions that can arise.

Chapter 5

Living with spastic diplegia

> Nobody gets to live life backward.
> Look ahead—that's where your future lies.
>
> **Ann Landers**

In this chapter, people share stories of living with spastic diplegia.

Melanie, mother of eight-year-old twins Cade and Graham, from Kentucky, US

"No wonder the heartbeat is so strong—there's TWO of them in there!"

Those were the words of the ultrasound tech one snowy morning. I had a positive pregnancy test the week before, and because I was spotting, my OB-GYN decided it would be best to see what was going on. Our first pregnancy had ended in a miscarriage; the second brought us our beautiful baby girl, Millie.

Nine-month-old Millie was sitting on my husband's lap during the ultrasound to see if our baby—BABIES—would be okay. That day set the tone for the rest of my pregnancy with our boys, Cade and Graham. After just a few months of biweekly appointments with the maternal-fetal medicine specialist, nonstop bleeding, and three trips to three different emergency rooms because I thought I was miscarrying, I went into labor at 24 weeks.

I was admitted to the hospital, and the providers were able to stop the labor. Then I went into labor again, and again it was stopped. The second time, however, my water broke, so when labor began a third time, at 25 weeks, the boys were delivered during an emergency C-section on July 6, 2015. I remember everyone in the OR being silent when both boys cried—they said at 25 weeks babies simply don't have the lung capacity to cry. My husband was able to hold the twins briefly after they were wrapped in plastic bags and blankets and before they were whisked away to the NICU.

Everything after that was a blur.

Cade and Graham were born a couple of minutes after 10:00 on a Monday morning, and at 4:30 a.m. the next day, the NICU doctor was in my room telling me both boys had collapsed lungs and had developed pneumonia, and that he didn't expect either one to make it through the day. They did make it, but a few days later, MRIs showed they both had bilateral brain bleeds.

Over the next few weeks, it felt like the boys were competing in a race: one would show a grade II brain bleed in the next MRI, and the other would say, "I see your grade II and raise you to a grade III," until both had maxed out at grade IV bleeds on both sides.

On really bad days, I wasn't allowed to hold either of the boys. On really, really bad days, the hospital chaplain visited them. For a while, we lived minute to minute. The NICU doctors prepared us for the worst-case scenario if the boys were ever discharged from the hospital. I remember one of the nurses, after a particularly brutal conversation with a doctor about the boys' capabilities in the future, reminding me to never limit our boys, no matter what the doctors say. Eight years later, I still hold those words close to my heart. They gave me hope in that moment and continued to do so through every physical therapy session, IEP meeting, doctor's appointment, and surgery.

About a month after the twins were born, their medical issues became too much for the level 3 NICU they were in, so they were transferred to a level 4 NICU in the same city. They each had three surgeries before becoming NICU graduates on October 28, 2015, two weeks after their due date. At first we thought we were in the clear when their first post-NICU checkups showed no signs of cerebral palsy. But when days and months passed and they missed developmental milestones, it came as no surprise to get their official diagnoses when they were two years old.

In those early days, we always had people alongside us, preparing us for the time we would need to make important decisions about the boys' medical interventions. One was their physical therapist who worked in Kentucky's Early Intervention System for children from birth to age three, who told us about different medications and procedures she had seen in her decades of experience, and offered advice on why some of them may not work for Cade and Graham, but others would. That background has allowed us to be better informed as we continue to navigate the health, education, and social systems to maximize opportunities for our boys.

To tell the stories of Cade and Graham is to also share with others their hearts. They are warriors and have had to fight to survive since day one. There has been no easy road for either of them. I couldn't tell you how many surgeries they've been through to this point, or even exactly how many diagnoses each boy has without pulling up their electronic medical records. But neither are angry or display jealousy of what other typical kids can do. Graham loves sports and remembers all the details from every event he's watched. (He may even be a little spoiled when he gets to announce batters at baseball and softball games.) Cade has a super-sweet connection to music: he can find his beat and match pitch and put all his heart into singing. Both of them are genuinely loving, trusting, resilient, and happy little boys.

So yes, that strong heartbeat the ultrasound tech heard tells the story of our boys, and there are TWO strong heartbeats. I'm so grateful that's true.

Jean, mother of nine-year-old William, from Ireland

William is an identical twin born in 2015 at 30 weeks gestation. The early birth was caused by twin-to-twin transfusion syndrome. The first diagnosis—of profound hearing loss—came within a few weeks of William's birth thanks to the national screening program that has been in place since 2011 in Ireland. In contrast, his diagnosis of cerebral palsy (spastic diplegia) wasn't made until he was almost three years old after continuing to fail his developmental milestones.

As his mother, I found it less daunting dealing with William's deafness after the initial shock of the diagnosis as I had a background in teaching children with speech and language disorders. A number of charity groups provided immediate support and information on the treatment pathway, working in cooperation with the National Hearing Implant Centre where William had his implant done, and connected us to a welcoming and supportive network of families with a similar diagnosis. Subsequently, accessing auditory verbal therapy, which was not widely available at the time, proved critical for William to develop typical speech and language ability.

Managing William's cerebral palsy diagnosis was a very different experience. Because cerebral palsy is a one-off injury to the brain, it is essential to exploit to the maximum the brain's plasticity in childhood by early intervention. Therefore, early diagnosis and provision of comprehensive information are the basic minimums in giving every child and their families a fighting chance for best outcomes.

Unfortunately, in our case, we felt alone and isolated, with no long-term treatment pathway being offered by the health service and little information available on how to move forward. In fact, a frequent sentiment we encountered was that we should keep our expectations low for William and accept how he was rather than be informed and educated about how he could reach his full potential.

We soon realized that we had to become the explorers and managers of William's treatment, and we turned to every information source we could find to plot a way forward. Thankfully, the power of the Internet to both inform us and connect to other families with CP in Ireland and abroad, and their willingness to advise and signpost us on this journey, was the game changer.

It was through contact with parents in Ireland, the UK, and Australia that we learned about SDR surgery, which William had in the US in April 2019. After his surgery, we embarked on regular five-day intensive physiotherapy sessions in specialist centers in the UK (as none are available in Ireland), working with practitioners brought to Ireland by families to treat their children, and regularly attending intensive swimming sessions in both Spain and Ireland. Again, we found all these services through online research, group forums, and calls with parents willing to help.

William's next major milestone was SPML surgery which he had done in January 2022, again in the US. He is currently attending an orthotic center in the UK for gait support using AFOs, which he wears to school.

Today, William rides his bike and scooter, trains with the local swimming club, practices Brazilian jiujitsu, plays mini-rugby in the winter and Gaelic football and hurling in the summer, and has clawed his way to the top of the mountains in County Clare where his great-grandmother's goats once roamed. He sings, plays the tin whistle, and enjoyed earning his first "income" last year while busking with his brothers at the Fleadh Cheoil, Ireland's national traditional music festival.

William's journey is by no means over—it is just beginning—and we must continue to learn about and prepare him for the treatment pathways through adolescence and into adulthood.

Edel, mother of nine-year-old Rossa, from Ireland

My son Rossa loves the rain. I share his joy in the wildness and the relentlessness nature of driving weather, especially by the sea—the wild Atlantic waves crashing, the rhythmic ebbs and flows, furiously pushing forcefully through any boundaries in its path. It is futile to try to impress on Rossa the merits of putting up a hood, as he will laugh uncontrollably and flick it off. He embraces the magical feeling that appeals to all the senses, reminding me (and perhaps himself subliminally), that he, too, is a force of nature, unstoppable and mighty.

Following an uneventful pregnancy, my second son was born without complication. We saw many beautiful cognitive milestones in the first few months, but physical milestones and irregularities began to haunt my inner thoughts and fears. Following an MRI at 11 months, a loose diagnosis of development delay was given, which later was interpreted as cerebral palsy. Rossa had SDR at age four and a half and progressed well after the operation. Unfortunately, a seizure disorder presented when he was five and a half, and things became less predictable as we navigated through various medications.

Rossa was—and is—my perfection. On the day of that MRI, after having had "the talk" from the consultant, I sat in the back seat of the car beside Rossa. I searched into his little face of 11 months old. He looked back at me with his usual wide-eyed glee, and I *knew*. Nothing any worried and woeful conversation with a doctor could shake that. Despite the clinical findings, I just *knew* our magical journey was going to continue just as it had begun. Like the wild Atlantic waves—unstoppable and mighty.

After the diagnosis, we set upon the pathway immediately toward therapeutic early intervention—a vast (albeit fruitful) minefield. Not every therapy regime fits every personal circumstance: the arduous strengthening sessions, the gentler play-based sensory input workouts, the swimming hydrotherapy, the hippotherapy, to name a few. Each intervention has a different effect and depends on the age and stage of the child. What works today may not be as effective tomorrow. To give each intervention a fair try can leave a family spinning. We found the best approach was to keep an open mind and be flexible to change things up as required.

As life went in a different direction physically for Rossa, we made a firm decision as a family to stay positive. There were choices on the table. One was getting swallowed up with the fear and dread. The other was to cut out negativity from the beginning and make our own pathway forward. This is indeed not an easy task. Handing over that precious time to worry and sleepless nights is challenging at times, but what could that ever achieve?

Instead, we keep a keen eye on having fun and living life as the priorities. Negativity would only serve as a disfavor to us all, but most importantly to Rossa. We made a conscious decision to move forward on our terms with our new reality each and every day as it unfolded for us. We were determined not to lose time that could be spent making magic memories as a family. This loss would only hamper our success, inner peace, and ultimate happiness. And in our family, Rossa stands out as the one who has understood this best. I look to him for strength sometimes and, unknowingly, he fills me up. We need him so much more than he needs us.

Rossa is naturally full of fun. Indeed, the Irish term "divilment," describes him perfectly: playfully mischievous. He is the middle of our three boys, who are close to each other in age, and with his innate story-telling ability and turn of phrase, he leaves people laughing hysterically with a hint of bemusement, as though they didn't see it coming. He is also an insatiable flirt with a mop of red curls. With a head turn and a laugh he knows that he is loved by many who need him at least as much as he needs them. These are the things that define him; his physical struggles do not.

That is not to underestimate the difficulties my son has faced and continues to face. It is more an explanation of the way life has carried us to the point we are at now. Of course, we do have our down days when things have become complicated, but by no means have these days defined us.

What challenges me the most when trying to navigate through a complicated and overburdened health system is that I will not rest until every possibility for positive change in my son has been explored and done so on a timely basis. It can be difficult to find a team who will give the commitment (and openness) to ongoing and timely investigation. My expectations are high but so are the stakes.

But as a family, we believe in hope and positivity and commitment to hard work, strength of character and resolve. Rossa shoulders the burden of this and yet finds time to quip at all of us, cutting us down to size with a merciless one-liner followed by a belly laugh. Like those who interact regularly with him, we take our lead from him.

Someone once asked me, "Did you ever think [as a mother], why me?" The negative implication of the question was not lost on me, but I answered from my heart: "Yes, I think that every day. How did I get to be the chosen one? I suppose that's just massive luck."

Of course, like every parent, I don't want Rossa to endure any struggle in life. But that is not the essence of my son. I am no different than any other mother wanting the best for her child and striving to be his voice when he needs it. I'm not naturally a particularly confident person, but I have steely confidence in my son and in his abilities to shine through life, and that is what leads me.

Many years ago, while on a trip to the UK for therapy, I found a little souvenir with a phrase that characterizes my little boy and our pathway: "Life isn't about waiting for the storm to pass, it is about learning to dance in the rain." We keep this visible in our home as it speaks to our family and reminds us how privileged we are.

Aaron, age 19, from Texas, US

My name is Aaron Jacob Navarro, and I am writing this to tell you about my experiences and advice for living with cerebral palsy.

I am currently going to college for business and working toward getting a job as a phlebotomist. I am also working part time at a convenience store. Sometimes that job is tough because I don't get to sit a lot and I'm on my feet most of my shift. My hobby right now is powerlifting. I compete in raw powerlifting and am working toward having an all-time world record in the open class one day. Later this year, I will compete in junior worlds for powerlifting in bench press. I want to show others that regardless of what sport or endeavor you choose, you can be great at just about anything you put your mind to.

I am saying these things to directly contradict the information that comes up when you google "cerebral palsy." There is a lot of scary and negative information on the Internet, but there are many different factors when it comes to cerebral palsy that counter some of that information. For the most part, I find what is said on the Internet about cerebral palsy and my condition to be far from the truth. I think that having cerebral palsy does not in any way mean you cannot live a long, happy life, or play a sport, or have fun hobbies.

If there's any advice I could give someone who is struggling with cerebral palsy, especially someone younger, it's that your happiness and success comes down to two things: attitude and work ethic.

Attitude: I will never forget the day that I was being rolled into my physical therapy session in a wheelchair after having SEMLS. I did not want to have another surgery and wondered if my life was ever going to be anything more than getting cut up over and over again.

Sitting in the PT room I could hear loud music being played right next to me. After looking around the corner, I saw a young boy who was in a wheelchair with little control of any of his limbs dancing. He was moving back and forth in his chair and moving his arms as much as he possibly could to dance. The best part was that he was laughing the whole time. I have met plenty of people who are much less happy. It was not until recently that I have come to realize no matter how upset others may be around me, I can and will be the happiest person in the room. When I was young, the doctors told my mother that I may never walk or that I would always have issues with walking. Now I deadlift and squat more than could be imagined. I continue to defy the doctors and push toward being better. That is the attitude you must have with cerebral palsy. Work hard toward proving the odds are wrong. Be kind, be positive, and maybe just a bit more hardheaded than anyone in the room.

Work ethic: Just because I was born with different legs doesn't mean I can't be a great bencher. Just because another kid has arms with spasticity, doesn't mean they can't be a great track runner. If you have bad motor pattern or use a wheelchair, who's to say you can't be valedictorian at your school, or get your master's degree and earn a six-figure salary someday. I'd rather be the kid with cerebral palsy who works harder than everyone than just "fit in" and be "normal." Normal is lame. Normal is average. Those of us who have a disability are not average; we are extraordinary. We have to work so much harder, and have so much grit. Don't ever let anyone make you a statistic or put limitations on what you can accomplish. Don't let people who make fun of you bother you too much either. They simply don't know anything about you or your condition. And please, please, stretch, and if you can, incorporate strength training into your life. Who knows where I would be if I had just stretched 30 minutes a day consistently when I was younger. Whether it's with bands, yoga, or a physical therapist, please stretch multiple times a week. I think it will do as much, if not more, good in some cases than any procedure can, and maybe even prevent some procedures. Another thing is to not worry too much about dating or breakups. Eventually, you will find someone who truly likes you for you.

Lastly, I hope if you only remember one thing from me it's this: keep moving forward until you reach your final goal, which is to be the best version of yourself you can possibly be, to prove wrong anyone who tells you can't do something along the path of life, to be kind to everyone, and to be your own hero.

Jessica, an adult, from Ireland

I was born in 1995, three months premature and weighing two pounds. This resulted in my diagnosis of spastic diplegic cerebral palsy, which affects mainly my legs and to a smaller degree my upper body. When I was a child, my parents would describe me as being very stubborn, determined, and independent. I walked using a walking frame, but also sometimes independently and often, as a child, wearing high heels (or as I called them, "hee highs") despite the disapproval of my physiotherapist.

Having a diagnosis of spastic diplegic cerebral palsy has shaped my life in many positive ways. The obstacles I faced filled me with curiosity and fueled me to study psychology and clinical neuroscience at university. With that foundation, I am currently enjoying a career as a researcher in CP.

Growing up with CP came with some great experiences. One was participating in para sports such as sailing, table tennis, wheelchair basketball, and horse riding. I even got to perform at the RDS (Royal Dublin Society) Horse Show once. I especially enjoyed traveling to many places I had never been to before to compete in different sport events, and meeting people like me I could relate to.

However, having CP has not been all joyful experiences. I was about 11 years old when I started to lose my ability to walk, eventually becoming fully dependent on my wheelchair. This had a significant impact on my mental health, particularly during adolescence. It was difficult for me to accept myself as my physical abilities changed. I experienced an array of emotions that I couldn't make sense of or even recognize at the time.

Adolescence is a difficult time for many people—with or without a disability—and many people experience mental illness, but I felt alone in my own experience as a young person with CP. The conversation and research about mental health challenges in people with CP has emerged only in recent years.

My lived experience led me to pursue a university degree with a goal to improve psychological supports and recognition for people like me. But that wasn't a smooth path, either, some of the time. Studying in third level didn't come easily to me. I found it difficult to concentrate and often experienced fatigue. I had to work extra hard compared to my peers. But I persevered, and my curiosity and passion to understand the potential impacts of having CP on psychological health were enough for me to succeed and progress to postgraduate studies (master of arts in psychology and master of science in clinical neuroscience).

Having CP has helped me stand out from the crowd in contributing to discussions and conducting research in a meaningful way in academia and now in my research career. It has all been a journey of self-discovery, one that helped me to understand myself and my emotions, which in turn helped me to accept myself and give me a great sense of healing, happiness, and excitement for my future.

Even though the journey with CP is a difficult one, I have learned that it is through these obstacles that you can find your purpose in life. Without my CP, I would not have been able to achieve everything I have today. Now that I'm an adult, whenever I am struggling emotionally or physically, I remember all I've accomplished and know I can overcome and achieve anything.

Ashley, an adult, from North Carolina, US

I would be lying if I said that living with cerebral palsy has never made my life difficult. In many ways, it absolutely has. I would also be lying if I said that living with cerebral palsy has made my life exceptional. It hasn't.

When you're born with a disability, you are often given—by way of existing societal tropes—two narrative options: either rise above the tragedy or lean into the "specialness" and the exceptionality.

After 31 years, I've realized that to live as a disabled person is to live in a way that is much more nuanced than most of the world will ever be able to realize or capture. I have been asked, more than once, what my parents did or didn't do for me that managed to make all the difference. They, of course, didn't get every single thing exactly right. Living in rural North Carolina in the pre-Internet age, they made the best possible use of the information and resources available to them. What they didn't do was make excuses for me or apologize for me or the things I needed—not ever. They made sure that I learned to ask for what I needed without shame, and that I had full permission to take up all the space I needed, never making myself smaller for the convenience of anyone. They made sure I knew that while they were always in my corner, my best advocate would always be my own self. Like I said, they maybe didn't get it all right all the time, but they tried really, really hard. And in my book (which, I think is the only book that counts here), they were pretty close to perfect.

I now work in the disability space professionally. I took a bit of a roundabout way of getting here, through publishing and graduate school and practicing as a speech-language pathologist. Despite that, I always hoped I would end up right where I am: writing, speaking, educating on disability and ableism, and as a nice surprise, directing adult research and programs at the Cerebral Palsy Foundation here in the US.

At a recent work meeting, we were having a conversation about the importance of maternal and prenatal care in reducing the incidence and prevalence of cerebral palsy. Right then, in a meeting room at a PR agency in New York City, I had a revelation: my cerebral palsy could have been completely and totally prevented if an OB-GYN had simply offered my mother an exploratory ultrasound after she experienced a miscarriage with twins in the spring of the year before I was born. Many people don't have a clue what caused their cerebral palsy, or maybe they have an incomplete answer, or maybe even just a guess. I have always known, though. Two words: septate uterus. As I grew to about 27 weeks gestation, I began putting pressure on the interior wall of my mom's divided uterus, which caused a silent placental abruption, early labor, and a very premature birth. It was during all the emergent panic of my birth that the uterine defect was discovered and removed. As a result, my younger sister was born at term, and without a trace of the palsy! Today she's an avid skier, surfer, and mountain biker. We like to joke that I paved the way for her to be such an outdoorswoman!

What I realized during that work meeting is how a simple ultrasound could have resulted, for better or worse, in an entirely different life for me. A life that I'm not entirely sure that I would want but certainly do think about sometimes. I think about it when I have so much neck tension that it turns into a migraine. When my feet hurt immediately after they hit the floor when I get up in the morning. When I'm in the grocery store, minding my business among the varieties of kale and get hit with, "Why do you walk like that?" or "What's wrong with you?" tossed casually out of the mouth of a stranger. When I think about all the ways that my own disability will undoubtedly leave a mark on my daughter's life. When I wish I could just *enjoy* the simple act of going for a walk in the sunshine.

I asked my husband one time and one time only: "Do you ever wish I didn't have CP?"

Whew, talk about a loaded question.

As usual, he didn't miss a beat: "No, because then you would be an entirely different person. You wouldn't be you."

I think that's the crux of it right there: I wouldn't choose a different, or easier, or less ableist, or whatever you want to call it kind of life.

In the world of disability, you hear the word "pride" a lot, and rightfully so. Each year in July as disability pride month comes around again and those conversations rise to the forefront, I always have complicated feelings. It feels a little uncomfortable for me to say that I am proud of my disability in and of itself. It feels strange and maybe even a little dishonest to say that I feel proud of the result of oxygen deprivation to my brain, an event I had literally nothing to do with.

What I *am* proud of is the life I live with cerebral palsy. Not the life I live in spite of it—no—but the life I live because of it.

Embracing this big, very obvious part of my life and identity, something that is simultaneously so visible and yet so nuanced, *that* is what I am so proud of. It has been quite the trip to get to this kind of acceptance. Not necessarily acceptance of the disability, for that has always been there, and I truly do not know any different, but the true and abiding acceptance of myself. I no longer worry about asking for what I need. I no longer worry about taking up space. And finally, after many, many years, I no longer give a single thought to how I am perceived by others *when* I walk into a room, all because of *how* I do it. Those perceptions are truly no longer a concern of mine.

Rachel, an adult, from Minnesota, US

As an adult in my 60s I am grateful to have the resources to lead an independent and productive life, even though I was born six weeks early in the late 1950s in rural Minnesota. My preterm birth resulted in spastic diplegia, which primarily affects my walking and balance. I was an independent ambulator until my mid-50s, at which time I started using walking sticks in the community, finding them more practical than crutches.

There are several reasons why I have a successful and fulfilling life. First and foremost is the love and support of my family and friends. I have always known that there were many people in my corner, and I have always tried to pay forward their generosity. My formal education has included bachelor's, master's, and doctoral degrees as well as several professional certifications. I am a lifelong learner both inside and outside the classroom. I have continuously been employed in positions I am passionate about, serving in senior leadership roles in government, higher education, health care, and the nonprofit sector. I currently serve as a fundraising professional for True Friends, an organization that provides experiences and adventures for people of all abilities.

I have been able to develop routines that support my lifestyle. I regularly work with a personal trainer, physical therapist, and massage therapist, and have been doing so consistently for the past 20 years. These professionals have provided me with excellent advice to help me pursue my goals and ensure I maintain the discipline of regular exercise.

In addition to working full time, I have many interests. I am actively involved in my community, and I travel internationally. I manage my own home and maintain an active social life, which includes my friend Bob, a gifted artist and entrepreneur who has survived a stroke. Our walking pace is such that we can keep up with each other.

I have been fortunate to live relatively pain-free. I had some back issues in my late 20s and early 30s that prompted me to discover Pilates and massage, which have largely erased the problems. I experienced some knee pain in my mid-50s. Traditional and specialized medical professionals were quick to say that it was a result of my CP; I needed to advocate for myself and not be satisfied that blaming my CP for acute issues would become a way of life for me. As it turned out, my knee pain was due to osteoarthritis. I had successful knee replacement surgery, which eliminated the knee pain. One point to note: the post-surgery rehabilitation took longer than would typically be expected for this type of surgery. I regained the ability to walk after the surgery, and my clinician now uses me as an example at international conferences of successful interventions in older adults.

When dealing with problems, I have found the following to be useful: persistence, patience, "out-of-the-box" problem-solving, and remembering that what might look like a "no" is merely a "not yet" or a "not this way."

My advice to a younger person is to remember that you are your own best advocate. I believe in taking the best information and professional advice and doing your best to make it work for you. Frequently, well-meaning individuals wanted me to direct my efforts toward disability. A vocational rehabilitation counselor suggested I abandon my pursuit of a degree in political science and change schools to become a vocational rehabilitation counselor. I ignored his question, "What would you ever do with a degree in political science?" In fact, my first job out of college was working for the governor of Minnesota. I found someone to make me custom boots that provided great support for my ankle and foot but were also stylish and functional; they did a lot to boost my self-confidence as a young adult.

My advice to readers of this book is to remember that this is just one point in time. The field of gait and motion management, physical therapy, and rehabilitation continues to change and advance. Be willing to inquire, suggest, and advocate for yourself. You may be a changemaker for yourself and many others.

I am a proud advocate for individuals with disabilities. Recently, my work and volunteerism have been well recognized in publications, including in *The New York Times* and the book *Pure Grit, Stories of Remarkable People Living with Physical Disability,* and by receiving the Corbett Ryan Pathways Pioneer Award given by the American Academy for Cerebral Palsy and Developmental Medicine.

Living with spastic diplegia plays a big part in my successes. Living with this condition has helped me to develop a broader and bolder vision, ignite my creativity, and embrace a willingness to persevere toward a desired outcome. I believe that my diagnosis is one aspect of my personhood that makes me fully human.

Chapter 6

Further reading and research

> Education is not the filling of a pail, but the lighting of a fire.
>
> **William Butler Yeats**

Further reading

For those who would like further reading on this condition, a list of recommended books, websites, and resources has been collated and will be regularly updated. Access to the list is provided in **Useful web resources.**

Research

Research serves as a cornerstone of evidence-based medicine and drives health care advancement. We discussed the importance of evidence-based medicine (or evidence-based practice) in Chapter 3. It is "the conscientious, explicit, and judicious use of current best evidence in making decisions about the care of individual patients." It combines the best available external clinical evidence from research with the clinical expertise of the professional.[169] Family priorities and preferences are also considered.[170]

Evidence is collected by carrying out scientific studies (research studies), the results of which are published as full-length, peer-reviewed research articles (or papers) in scientific journals. "Peer-reviewed" means that experts with relevant content knowledge have reviewed, challenged, and agreed that the scientific method and study conclusions based on the results are sound.

Scientific studies may also be presented in brief at conferences, and conference proceedings are often published. However, conference proceedings present preliminary results and peer review is minimal. *Therefore, full-length published research articles are the most rigorous and sound evidence.*

The above published research outputs are collectively known as scientific literature or, simply, research.

Research may also be discussed on various social media platforms such as X (formerly Twitter), Facebook, LinkedIn, and Instagram. If you consume information this way, it is always important to go back to the original source (i.e., the full-length research article) to ensure the media's portrayal of the study findings is accurate.

You may have familiarity with searching the scientific literature. If not, search engines such as PubMed (ncbi.nlm.nih.gov/pubmed) and Google Scholar (scholar.google.com) are good places to start. They provide a free abstract (a short summary of the article), which can be very useful. In the past, you generally needed to belong to an academic or medical institution to have access to full-length research articles. Many articles are now available online for free. Google Scholar provides links to many full-length articles, and some community libraries allow you to request full-length articles.

You might have heard the phrase, "Just because someone says it, doesn't mean it's true." This is worth remembering in all aspects of life, but it is also relevant to research. While research articles go through a peer review process, you should still read them with a critical eye. Ask yourself, How confident can I be in the results of this research study? Was the sample size big enough to be representative of the larger population? Did the results support the conclusion?

If you aren't a trained scientist, reviewing the quality of the evidence might be more challenging, but you can still make sure the basic methods make sense and the author's conclusions are supported by the data presented. The information below will help you learn about some research study designs and how study design affects how much confidence you can place in a study's conclusions.

Research study design

There are different research study designs, and each has its value. The quality of the evidence, or level of evidence, is graded based on the study design and how well the methods were executed. Research articles sometimes list (often in the abstract) the level of evidence from I to V, with level I being the highest.

The most common research study designs, listed from highest to lowest level of evidence, are:

* Systematic review
* Randomized controlled trial
* Cohort
* Case control
* Cross-sectional
* Case report and case series

Systematic review: A systematic review summarizes the results of several scientific studies on the same topic. They can be qualitative (descriptive) or quantitative (numerical):

* Qualitative: A summary of common themes and findings across studies but without a statistical analysis.
* Quantitative: A statistical analysis carried out that takes a weighted average of the findings across studies to produce one estimate for the effect of a treatment, for example. The quantitative approach is called a "meta-analysis."

The highest level of evidence is a systematic review of randomized controlled trials (described next), although systematic reviews can also include studies that used other types of study designs. Systematic reviews may be published by individual researchers or groups. The Cochrane collaboration is a worldwide association of researchers, health care professionals, patients, and carers that publishes systematic reviews on various topics.

Randomized controlled trial (RCT): An RCT is a study design aimed at identifying cause and effect. The cause is, for example, the treatment, and the effect is the outcome being measured. Strict control of the study method (the "C" in RCT) helps to ensure the treatment of interest is the only factor that could cause the outcome. A treatment group receives the treatment while a nontreatment group (also known as the control group) does not. The participants are randomly assigned (the "R" in RCT) to one of the groups. The random assignment is one of the key strengths of this study design because it takes care of the "unknown unknowns" that may influence the outcome. The treatment effect is found by comparing the outcomes of the treatment and nontreatment groups. RCTs are considered the highest quality study design but are still uncommon in medical literature.

Cohort: A cohort is a group of people who share a common characteristic (e.g., diagnosis, gender). In a cohort study, outcome is measured two or more times. Researchers identify the characteristic of interest and then measure the outcome, looking for associations between the two. A cohort study is a form of longitudinal study ("longitudinal" means that the same outcome is measured on the same participants two or more times over a period of time). You may come across the terms "prospective" and "retrospective" cohort studies.

- In prospective cohort studies, research questions and methods are defined, and a cohort is followed over time, collecting data.
- In retrospective cohort studies, research questions and methods are defined after data has been collected or already exists (e.g., a person's medical record).

Case control: In case control studies, researchers identify the outcome of interest, which defines the groups (e.g., infants with a specific diagnosis and typically developing infants), and then look backward in time at different factors or exposures that might have caused different outcomes. At the beginning of the study, the outcome is known, but the factors or exposures that might have caused that outcome are unknown. This is the opposite of cohort studies. Because the outcome and factors or exposures data already exist, case control studies are always retrospective.

Cross-sectional: Cross-sectional studies take measurements only once from participants. Researchers look for associations between certain factors and exposures, and outcomes.

Case report and case series: A case report (also referred to as a single-subject case study) is an account of a single patient—usually a unique case—and their medical history, status, and outcomes from a treatment, for example. A case series is a group of case reports on patients who were exposed to a similar treatment. These reports are usually retrospective, and data has already been collected by other means (usually as part of routine medical care).

Getting involved in research

There are many opportunities to become involved in research. Together with medical professionals and researchers, people with lived experience can help drive advancement in health care.

a) As a participant

Researchers working in academic and medical settings are always looking for participants for their studies. You might receive an invitation to participate in such a study via an email, letter in the mail, phone call, social media ad, or other method.

Some studies are very easy and may just involve completing one online survey; others may take more time with various measurements being taken on more than one occasion. Just as you are advised to read published research studies with a critical eye, so should you judge new research study opportunities before agreeing to participate. Participating can take time and effort—the expected time commitment will be communicated in the study recruitment material. There is often a small reimbursement offered for time spent in a study.

It's worth noting that you, as the study participant, may not personally benefit from the research study, but the collective population with the condition will likely benefit.

Clinical trials are research studies conducted to evaluate the safety and effectiveness of new medical treatments, including new medications and devices before they can be approved for widespread use. They are often conducted following a randomized controlled trial research study design.

A potential benefit of participating in clinical trials is gaining early access to new medical treatments. Even if you are assigned to the control group (which usually receives standard care), you may have early access to the new treatment once the data collection phase is complete. In addition, standard care is likely to be current best practice.

You can find information about clinical trials through various sources:

- The National Institutes of Health in the US maintains a comprehensive database, ClinicalTrials.gov, where you can learn about clinical trials around the world. You can search this database by specific medical condition, location, or other pertinent criteria to identify relevant clinical trials that may be currently enrolling participants.
- Major academic medical centers, research institutions, and hospitals often conduct clinical trials and can provide information about their ongoing studies.
- Medical professionals may be aware of ongoing clinical trials in their field and can provide guidance to families who are interested in participating.
- Organizations that support particular conditions are another source of information.

Depending on the nature of the treatment in the clinical trial, you may want to, or be required to, consult with your medical professional to help you consider the risks and benefits of participating.

b) As a co-producer

Family engagement in research (FER) plays a crucial role in fostering collaboration and helping improve study design and outcome. When families become involved in research as collaborators on a study rather than simply as participants, researchers gain valuable insights into the lived experiences and perspectives of families. Families participate at every stage of the research process: concept, design, planning, conduct, and reporting of the study findings. These opportunities are still rare but are becoming more common. As an example, a link to the FER program at Gillette Children's is included in **Useful web resources**.

The family engagement in research movement is largely attributed to the similar and earlier patient and public involvement initiative in the UK. Here are some opportunities:

- **CanChild** and the **Kids Brain Health Network** in Canada currently offer The Family Engagement in Research program, a short online training course through McMaster University Continuing Education, to train family members and researchers (including coordinators and assistants) in collaborating on research.
- Online training modules are available at **Patient-Oriented Research Curriculum in Child Health (PORCCH)**.
- The **Patient-Centered Outcomes Research Institute (PCORI)** and the **Strategy for Patient-Oriented Research (SPOR)** are two other organizations that encourage family engagement.

Epilogue

You see things; and you say "Why?"
But I dream things that never were;
and I say "Why not?"
George Bernard Shaw

I'll leave the last words to Tommy.

For as long as I can remember, I've thought most clearly while writing. When I was a teenager, I kept a blog and wrote about 1,200 posts in the space of three years. I wrote about everything and nothing at all: the classes I was taking at school, the books I was reading, the latest Broadway show I was obsessing about.

Growing up, I spent a lot of time thinking about how to be disabled without letting that one fact take over my life. As a teenager, I found it easiest to ignore my disability as much as I could. I wouldn't mention it, and people mostly did the same. I hated those moments when I couldn't ignore it—when I fell, when I got injured, or when I dropped something.

Of course, I couldn't ignore it entirely: large portions of my teenage years were consumed by joint pain and sleepless nights. I spent hours in physical therapy and had two major surgeries. When I was 18, I realized I wanted to write something about it. So over one summer, I holed myself up in my room and wrote a short book. It was autobiographical in the sense that it charted the various surgeries and treatments I'd had, but more than that, it allowed me to work through what it meant to be disabled. There's no user manual for having a disability, but I was trying to write the next best thing for myself. I named the book *Consider This*, in part because it was what I was doing (considering this disability, if you will), and in part because of a line in R.E.M.'s "Losing My Religion," one of my favorite songs.

I remember lying awake with joint pain one night in August that summer. I couldn't sleep, and, more annoyingly, I couldn't figure out how to finish the short book I'd written. I was about to start my last year of high school, and the narrative of the book ended a few months before that. On the one hand, it felt like a natural stopping point, but on the other, it still felt like the middle of the story. What had I learned writing the book? What would I take from it?

I got up and wrote a letter—a sort of what-I-wish-I'd-known letter to the Tommy of a decade ago. I wrote about how to keep a disability in perspective and concentrate on what actually matters in life. I framed it as the letter I'd write if I had a child with spastic diplegia. It became the epilogue to my short book; I've included it below.

A lot has changed in the years since I wrote that piece. I can't ignore the fact that I'm disabled, no matter how much I try (and I tried!). But I've gotten much better at knowing my own limitations and being comfortable enough to ask for help when I need it. Instead of staying quiet and struggling with something, I'm more comfortable around people, and I get more done.

I'm still missing the user manual for how to get through life with a disability. I'd write a very different book if I were starting it today, but I'm proud of how *Consider This* stands on its own.

When I was writing it, I had no idea that my mother would one day write a book about spastic diplegia. In a lot of ways, the two books are in conversation with one another across time. I hope *Consider This* is as useful for you to read as it was for me to write.

August 17, 2012

I owe everything I am today to my parents, so I can only hope to live up to half of what they are. They're the most loving, caring, and dedicated parents anyone could ask for, and I hope I can be the same to you. Having a disability is tough, but you can handle it. I did. It was hard—probably the hardest thing I've had to do—but I did it. And so can you. Some days it's unimaginably difficult to get out of bed and face the world, but it's possible.

So, how do you beat your disability? You beat it by never letting it define you. I wasn't a 14-year-old who had CP, I was a 14-year-old who loved drums, read every book he could lay his hands on, and probably played his music too loud. As people, we're defined not by our abilities or disabilities—it's our choices, our aspirations, and our attitudes that define us. So go out there and be outrageously passionate about something.

You beat your disability by knowing where you want to be—be that on crutches or walking independently—and then working your ass off to get there. You beat it by never settling for less than what you can achieve. You might have a disability, but don't let the disability have you.

You beat it by setting goals. I could quote life mottos like, "Don't wait for your ship to come in, swim out to meet it," but nobody listens to those. That said, they are rooted in truth. Managing your CP isn't something that's going to fall into your lap as you sit at home moping: you have to work toward it. You beat it with pragmatism. It's true, you'll probably never be a professional footballer. Or an astronaut. Or a stunt double. Or a boxer. You're faced with a choice: let yourself be constantly held back by it, or shrug it off and focus on all the things you can do.

And then, if you manage all that? You'll have beaten it—and, more importantly, you'll have the satisfaction of leading a full life despite your disability. And that's an incredible achievement.

—Tommy

Tommy's book is available at
www.GilletteChildrensHealthcarePress.org/sdbook.

Acknowledgments

It takes a village to raise a child

African proverb

And it takes a village to produce a Healthcare Series. Publication of this series began with an idea, then with five titles, and then more titles. These acknowledgments relate to the entire series.

The formula of deep medical information interspersed with lived experience gives readers an appreciation of the childhood-acquired, often lifelong conditions. We thank the many people who contributed to each title: medical professionals at Gillette Children's who willingly came forward to lead each book; Gillette writers who did the research and writing of each; other Gillette team members who contributed from their different specialties; family authors and vignette writers who shared their personal stories; other families who shared photographs; the Gillette editing team who ensured the content and structure worked for the reader; Olwyn Roche who beautifully illustrated each title; advance readers, both professionals and families, whose feedback was invaluable; and Lina Abdennabi who coordinated Gillette Press operations. Behind every book was also a pit team who converted the finished manuscript into the book you now hold. Ruth Wilson led and looked after copyediting and proofreading. Jazmin Welch created the beautiful design and layout. Audrey McClellan indexed each title.

Smoothly creating each title required great teamwork among our villagers.

Staff at Gillette Children's provided continual support to the project and everyone involved. This included the steering committee, in particular Paula Montgomery, Dr. Micah Niermann, and Barbara Joers.

This Healthcare Series is co-published with Mac Keith Press. From the get-go, the journey with Ann-Marie Halligan and Sally Wilkinson was one of great support and collaboration.

Gillette Children's Healthcare Press

Glossary

Grasp the subject, the words will follow.

Cato the Elder

TERM	DEFINITION
Abnormal/atypical	Deviating from the typical expectation.
Achilles tendon	The cord-like structure that attaches the gastrocnemius and soleus muscles (both calf muscles) to the bone at the heel.
Ankle-foot orthosis (AFO)	A type of orthosis (brace or splint) that controls the ankle and foot. See *orthosis*.
Baclofen	A medication used for tone reduction; can be delivered either orally or by using a pump connected to a catheter to deliver the medication to the intrathecal area (the fluid-filled space surrounding the spinal cord). The latter delivery method is called intrathecal baclofen (ITB).
Bilateral CP	A form of cerebral palsy that affects both sides of the body.
Botulinum neurotoxin A (BoNT-A)	A medication used for tone reduction. It is delivered by injection directly into the muscle.
Cardiometabolic	Referring to both heart disease and metabolic disorders (such as diabetes).
Casting	The process of stretching a muscle by applying a plaster of paris or a fiberglass cast; for example, a below-knee cast to stretch the tight gastrocnemius and/or soleus muscles (calf muscles) to hold the muscle in a position of maximum stretch.

Centers for Disease Control and Prevention (CDC)	The national public health institute in the US.
Cerebral	Referring to the cerebrum, the front and upper part of the brain, one of the major areas responsible for the control of movement.
Contracture	A limitation of the range of motion of a joint. It occurs in the muscle-tendon unit (MTU) and/or capsule of the joint, not just the muscle. See *muscle-tendon unit; range of motion.*
Crouch gait	A persistent flexed-knee gait. The exact degree of knee flexion that constitutes crouch gait varies in the literature but is typically greater than or equal to 20 degrees. This knee flexion is normally also accompanied by persistent hip flexion. The foot position can be variable. See *gait.*
Diplegia	A form of cerebral palsy affecting all limbs, but the lower limbs are much more affected than the upper limbs, which frequently show only fine motor impairment.
Dystonia	A condition characterized by involuntary muscle contractions that cause slow repetitive movements or abnormal postures that can sometimes be painful.
Episode of care (EOC)	A period of therapy (at the appropriate frequency) followed by a therapy break.
Fine motor function	Refers to the smaller movements in the wrists, hands, fingers, and toes. Examples include picking up objects between the thumb and forefinger, and writing. Also called fine motor skills, hand skills, fine motor coordination, or dexterity.
Gait	A person's manner of walking.
Gait analysis	A measurement tool used to evaluate gait. Within gait analysis, multiple variables are evaluated using different measurement tools.

Gross motor function	The ability to make large, general movement of the arms, legs, and other large body parts, such as sitting, crawling, standing, running, jumping, swimming, throwing, catching, and kicking. Also called gross motor skills.
Gross Motor Function Classification System (GMFCS)	A five-level classification system that describes the functional mobilities of children and adolescents with cerebral palsy. Level I has the fewest limitations and level V has the most. It provides an indication of the severity of cerebral palsy.
Hemiplegia	A form of cerebral palsy affecting the upper and lower limbs on one side of the body. The upper limb is usually more affected than the lower limb.
Hypotonia/hypertonia	See *muscle tone*.
International Classification of Functioning, Disability and Health (ICF)	A universal framework for considering any health condition. It helps show the impact of a health condition at different levels and how those levels are interconnected.
Magnetic resonance imaging (MRI)	A noninvasive imaging technology that produces detailed three-dimensional anatomical images without the use of radiation.
Muscle-tendon unit (MTU)	A combination of the muscle, tendon, and other structures.
Muscle tone	The resting tension in a person's muscles. Tone is considered abnormal when it falls outside the range of normal or typical; either too low (hypotonia) or too high (hypertonia). Abnormal muscle tone occurs in all types of cerebral palsy.
Musculoskeletal	Referring to both the muscles and the skeleton; includes muscles, bones, joints, and their related structures (e.g., ligaments, and tendons). The term *neuromusculoskeletal* includes the nervous system.
Neurology	Specialty dealing with disorders of the nervous system.
Neuromusculoskeletal	Referring to the nervous system, muscles, bones, joints, and their related structures.
Neurosurgery	Specialty that involves surgical management of disorders of the nervous system.

Occupational therapy	A type of therapy based on engaging in everyday activities (occupations) to promote health, well-being, and independence.
Orthopedic surgery	Specialty that involves surgical management of disorders affecting the *musculoskeletal* system.
Orthosis	A device designed to hold specific body parts in position to modify their structure and/or function; also called a brace or splint.
Orthotics	The branch of medicine concerned with the design, manufacture, and management of orthoses. See *orthosis.*
Osteoporosis	A medical condition where the bones are weak and brittle, with low density.
Palsy	Paralysis (though paralysis by pure definition is not a feature of cerebral palsy).
Pediatrics	Specialty dealing with children and their conditions.
Percentile	A variable (such as a person's height by age) that divides the distribution of the variable into 100 groups. The 50th percentile is always the median (the midpoint that separates lower and higher values into two groups).
Physiatry	See *physical medicine and rehabilitation.*
Physical medicine and rehabilitation (PM&R)	Specialty that aims to enhance and restore functional ability and quality of life among those with physical disabilities. Also termed *physiatry.*
Physical therapy/ physiotherapy	A type of therapy to develop, maintain, and restore a person's maximum movement and functional ability.
Quadriplegia	A form of cerebral palsy affecting all four limbs and the trunk; also known as tetraplegia.
Range of motion (ROM)	A measure of joint flexibility; the range through which a joint moves, measured in degrees. Also called range of movement.
Selective dorsal rhizotomy (SDR)	Refers to the selective cutting of abnormal sensory nerve rootlets in the spinal cord to reduce spasticity.

Single-event multilevel surgery (SEMLS)	Multiple orthopedic surgical procedures performed during a single operation.
Spasticity	A condition in which there is an abnormal increase in muscle tone or stiffness of muscle that can interfere with movement and speech, and be associated with discomfort or pain.
Speech and language pathology (SLP)	A type of therapy to support those with speech, language, and communication needs as well as feeding and swallowing difficulties. Also called speech and language therapy.
Tendon	The cord-like structure that attaches the muscle to the bone; for example, the *Achilles tendon* attaches both calf muscles to the bone at the heel.
Tone	See *muscle tone*.
Unilateral CP	A form of cerebral palsy that affects one side of the body.
W-sitting	A description of the sitting position often adopted by a child with cerebral palsy where the child's bottom is on the floor while their legs are out to each side; looking from the top, the legs form a "W" shape.

References

1.	World Health Organization (2001) *International classification of functioning, disability and health (ICF)*. [online] Available at: <https://www.who.int/standards/classifications/international-classification-of-functioning-disability-and-health> [Accessed February 22 2024].

2.	Rosenbaum P, Paneth N, Leviton A, et al. (2007) A report: The definition and classification of cerebral palsy April 2006. *Dev Med Child Neurol Suppl,* 109, 8–14.

3.	Graham HK, Rosenbaum P, Paneth N, et al. (2016) Cerebral palsy. *Nat Rev Dis Primers,* 2, 1–24.

4.	Smithers-Sheedy H, Waight E, Goldsmith S, McIntyre S (2023) Australian Cerebral Palsy Register report, Available at: <https://cpregister.com/wp-content/uploads/2023/01/2023-ACPR-Report.pdf> [Accessed June 24 2024].

5.	McIntyre S, Goldsmith S, Webb A, et al. (2022) Global prevalence of cerebral palsy: A systematic analysis. *Dev Med Child Neurol,* 64, 1494–1506.

6.	Centers for Disease Control and Prevention (2024a) *Epidemiology glossary.* [online] Available at: <https://www.cdc.gov/reproductive-health/glossary/> [Accessed June 24 2024].

7.	Shepherd E, Salam RA, Middleton P, et al. (2017) Antenatal and intrapartum interventions for preventing cerebral palsy: An overview of Cochrane systematic reviews. *Cochrane Database Syst Rev,* 8, 1–78.

8.	Rosenbaum P, Rosenbloom L (2012) *Cerebral palsy: From diagnosis to adult life,* London: Mac Keith Press.

9.	National Institute of Neurological Disorders and Stroke (2023a) *Cerebral palsy.* [online] Available at: <https://www.ninds.nih.gov/health-information/disorders/cerebral-palsy> [Accessed June 21 2024].

10.	Centers for Disease Control and Prevention (2024b) *Risk factors for cerebral palsy.* [online] Available at: <https://www.cdc.gov/cerebral-palsy/risk-factors/> [Accessed June 18 2024].

11.	Centers for Disease Control and Prevention (2017) *Single embryo transfer.* [online] Available at: <https://www.cdc.gov/art/patientresources/transfer.html> [Accessed June 24 2024].

12.	National Perinatal Epidemiology and Statistics Unit (2021) IVF success rates have improved in the last decade, especially in older women: Report, Australia, UNSW, Available at: <https://www.unsw.edu.au/newsroom/news/2021/09/ivf-success-rates-have-improved-in-the-last-decade--especially-i> [Accessed January 19 2024].

13.	Nelson KB (2008) Causative factors in cerebral palsy. *Clin Obstet Gynecol,* 51, 749–62.

14. Novak I, Morgan C, Fahey M, et al. (2020) State of the evidence traffic lights 2019: Systematic review of interventions for preventing and treating children with cerebral palsy. *Curr Neurol Neurosci Rep*, 20, 1–21.

15. Durkin MS, Benedict RE, Christensen D, et al. (2016) Prevalence of cerebral palsy among 8-year-old children in 2010 and preliminary evidence of trends in its relationship to low birthweight. *Paediatr Perinat Epidemiol*, 30, 496–510.

16. McGuire DO, Tian LH, Yeargin-Allsopp M, Dowling NF, Christensen DL (2019) Prevalence of cerebral palsy, intellectual disability, hearing loss, and blindness, National Health Interview Survey, 2009–2016. *Disabil Health J*, 12, 443–451.

17. Khandaker G, Muhit M, Karim T, et al. (2019) Epidemiology of cerebral palsy in Bangladesh: A population-based surveillance study. *Dev Med Child Neurol*, 61, 601–609.

18. Centers for Disease Control and Prevention (2024c) *Down syndrome.* [online] Available at: <https://www.cdc.gov/ncbddd/birthdefects/downsyndrome.html> [Accessed June 21 2024].

19. National Institutes of Health (2024) *Estimates of funding for various research, condition, and disease categories (RCDC).* [online] Available at: <https://report .nih.gov/funding/categorical-spending#/> [Accessed June 21 2024].

20. Mathew JL, Kaur N, Dsouza JM (2022) Therapeutic hypothermia in neonatal hypoxic encephalopathy: A systematic review and meta-analysis. *J Glob Health*, 12, 1–22.

21. Novak I, Morgan C, Adde L, et al. (2017) Early, accurate diagnosis and early intervention in cerebral palsy. *JAMA Pediatr*, 171, 1–11.

22. National Institute of Neurological Disorders and Stroke (2024) *Glossary of neurological terms.* [online] Available at: <https://www.ninds.nih.gov/health -information/disorders/glossary-neurological-terms> [Accessed June 14 2024].

23. Byrne R, Noritz G, Maitre NL, N.C.H. Early Developmental Group (2017) Implementation of early diagnosis and intervention guidelines for cerebral palsy in a high-risk infant follow-up clinic. *Pediatr Neurol*, 76, 66–71.

24. Maitre NL, Burton VJ, Duncan AF, et al. (2020) Network implementation of guideline for early detection decreases age at cerebral palsy diagnosis. *Pediatrics*, 145, 1–10.

25. Te Velde A, Tantsis E, Novak I, et al. (2021) Age of diagnosis, fidelity and acceptability of an early diagnosis clinic for cerebral palsy: A single site imple-mentation study. *Brain Sci*, 11, 1–14.

26. King AR, Machipisa C, Finlayson F, et al. (2021) Early detection of cerebral palsy in high-risk infants: Translation of evidence into practice in an Australian hospital. *J Paediatr Child Health*, 57, 246–250.

27. King AR, Al Imam MH, McIntyre S, et al. (2022) Early diagnosis of cerebral palsy in low- and middle-income countries. *Brain Sci*, 12, 1–13.

28. Maitre NL, Damiano D, Byrne R (2023) Implementation of early detection and intervention for cerebral palsy in high-risk infant follow-up programs: U.S. and global considerations. *Clin Perinatol*, 50, 269–279.

29. Maitre NL, Byrne R, Duncan A, et al. (2022) "High-risk for cerebral palsy" designation: A clinical consensus statement. *J Pediatr Rehabil Med*, 15, 165–174.

30. Morgan C, Fetters L, Adde L, et al. (2021) Early intervention for children aged 0 to 2 years with or at high risk of cerebral palsy: International clinical practice guideline based on systematic reviews. *JAMA Pediatr,* 175, 846–858.

31. Ismail FY, Fatemi A, Johnston MV (2017) Cerebral plasticity: Windows of opportunity in the developing brain. *Eur J Paediatr Neurol,* 21, 23–48.

32. Cerebral Palsy Alliance (2019) *Why neuroplasticity is the secret ingredient for kids with special needs.* [online] Available at: <https://cerebralpalsy.org.au/news-stories/why-neuroplasticity-is-the-secret-ingredient-for-kids-with-special-needs/> [Accessed June 14 2024].

33. Kohli-Lynch M, Tann CJ, Ellis ME (2019) Early intervention for children at high risk of developmental disability in low- and middle-income countries: A narrative review. *Int J Environ Res Public Health,* 16, 1–9.

34. McNamara L, Morgan C, Novak I (2023) Interventions for motor disorders in high-risk neonates. *Clin Perinatol,* 50, 121–155.

35. Byrne R, Duncan A, Pickar T, et al. (2019) Comparing parent and provider priorities in discussions of early detection and intervention for infants with and at risk of cerebral palsy. *Child Care Health Dev,* 45, 799–807.

36. Centers for Disease Control and Prevention (2024d) *CDC's developmental milestones.* [online] Available at: <https://www.cdc.gov/ncbddd/actearly/milestones/index.html> [Accessed June 21 2024].

37. WHO Multicentre Growth Reference Study Group (2006) WHO motor development study: Windows of achievement for six gross motor development milestones. *Acta Paediatr Suppl,* 450, 86–95.

38. Surveillance of Cerebral Palsy in Europe (2000) A collaboration of cerebral palsy surveys and registers. Surveillance of cerebral palsy in Europe (SCPE). *Dev Med Child Neurol,* 42, 816–24.

39. National Institute of Neurological Disorders and Stroke (2021) *Dystonia [pdf].* [online] Available at: <https://catalog.ninds.nih.gov/sites/default/files/publications/dystonia.pdf> [Accessed January 19 2024].

40. National Institute of Neurological Disorders and Stroke (2023b) *Ataxia and cerebellar or spinocerebellar degeneration.* [online] Available at: <https://www.ninds.nih.gov/health-information/disorders/ataxia-and-cerebellar-or-spinocerebellar-degeneration> [Accessed January 19 2024].

41. Centers for Disease Control and Prevention (2024e) *About cerebral palsy.* [online] Available at: <https://www.cdc.gov/cerebral-palsy/about/> [Accessed June 21 2024].

42. Australian Cerebral Palsy Register (2023) *Personal communication.*

43. Gorter JW, Rosenbaum PL, Hanna SE, et al. (2004) Limb distribution, motor impairment, and functional classification of cerebral palsy. *Dev Med Child Neurol,* 46, 461–7.

44. Himmelmann K, Beckung E, Hagberg G, Uvebrant P (2006) Gross and fine motor function and accompanying impairments in cerebral palsy. *Dev Med Child Neurol,* 48, 417–23.

45. Shevell MI, Dagenais L, Hall N, Repacq C (2009) The relationship of cerebral palsy subtype and functional motor impairment: A population-based study. *Dev Med Child Neurol,* 51, 872–7.

46. Hidecker MJ, Ho NT, Dodge N, et al. (2012) Inter-relationships of functional status in cerebral palsy: Analyzing Gross Motor Function, Manual Ability, and Communication Function Classification Systems in children. *Dev Med Child Neurol*, 54, 737–42.

47. Aravamuthan BR, Fehlings D, Shetty S, et al. (2021) Variability in cerebral palsy diagnosis. *Pediatrics*, 147, 1–11.

48. Dar H, Stewart K, McIntyre S, Paget S (2023) Multiple motor disorders in cerebral palsy. *Dev Med Child Neurol*, 66, 317–325.

49. Palisano R, Rosenbaum P, Walter S, et al. (1997) Development and reliability of a system to classify gross motor function in children with cerebral palsy. *Dev Med Child Neurol*, 39, 214–23.

50. Palisano RJ, Rosenbaum P, Bartlett D, Livingston MH (2008) Content validity of the expanded and revised Gross Motor Function Classification System. *Dev Med Child Neurol*, 50, 744–50.

51. Alriksson-Schmidt A, Nordmark E, Czuba T, Westbom L (2017) Stability of the Gross Motor Function Classification System in children and adolescents with cerebral palsy: A retrospective cohort registry study. *Dev Med Child Neurol*, 59, 641–646.

52. Huroy M, Behlim T, Andersen J, et al. (2022) Stability of the Gross Motor Function Classification System over time in children with cerebral palsy. *Dev Med Child Neurol*, 64, 1487–1493.

53. McCormick A, Brien M, Plourde J, et al. (2007) Stability of the Gross Motor Function Classification System in adults with cerebral palsy. *Dev Med Child Neurol*, 49, 265–9.

54. Kinsner-Ovaskainen A, Lanzoni M, Martin S, et al. (2017) *Surveillance of cerebral palsy in Europe: Development of the JRC-SCPE central database and public health indicators,* Luxembourg: Publications Office of the European Union.

55. Rosenbaum PL, Walter SD, Hanna SE, et al. (2002) Prognosis for gross motor function in cerebral palsy: Creation of motor development curves. *JAMA*, 288, 1357–63.

56. Hanna SE, Bartlett DJ, Rivard LM, Russell DJ (2008) Reference curves for the Gross Motor Function Measure: Percentiles for clinical description and tracking over time among children with cerebral palsy. *Phys Ther*, 88, 596–607.

57. Eliasson AC, Krumlinde-Sundholm L, Rösblad B, et al. (2006) The Manual Ability Classification System (MACS) for children with cerebral palsy: Scale development and evidence of validity and reliability. *Dev Med Child Neurol*, 48, 549–54.

58. Eliasson AC, Ullenhag A, Wahlstrom U, Krumlinde-Sundholm L (2017) Mini-MACS: Development of the Manual Ability Classification System for children younger than 4 years of age with signs of cerebral palsy. *Dev Med Child Neurol*, 59, 72–78.

59. Beckung E, Hagberg G (2002) Neuroimpairments, activity limitations, and participation restrictions in children with cerebral palsy. *Dev Med Child Neurol*, 44, 309–16.

60. Elvrum AK, Andersen GL, Himmelmann K, et al. (2016) Bimanual Fine Motor Function (BFMF) classification in children with cerebral palsy: Aspects of construct and content validity. *Phys Occup Ther Pediatr*, 36, 1–16.

61. Elvrum AG, Beckung E, Saether R, et al. (2017) Bimanual capacity of children with cerebral palsy: Intra- and interrater reliability of a revised edition of the Bimanual Fine Motor Function classification. *Phys Occup Ther Pediatr*, 37, 239–251.

62. Hidecker MJ, Paneth N, Rosenbaum PL, et al. (2011) Developing and validating the Communication Function Classification System for individuals with cerebral palsy. *Dev Med Child Neurol*, 53, 704–10.

63. Pennington L, Mjøen T, Da Graça Andrada M, Murray J (2010) Viking Speech Scale [pdf] EU, European Commission, Available at: <https://eu-rd-platform.jrc.ec.europa.eu/sites/default/files/Viking-Speech-Scale-2011-Copyright_EN.pdf> [Accessed June 18 2024].

64. Pennington L, Virella D, Mjøen T, et al. (2013) Development of the Viking Speech Scale to classify the speech of children with cerebral palsy. *Res Dev Disabil*, 34, 3202–10.

65. Virella D, Pennington L, Andersen GL, et al. (2016) Classification systems of communication for use in epidemiological surveillance of children with cerebral palsy. *Dev Med Child Neurol*, 58, 285–91.

66. Sellers D, Mandy A, Pennington L, Hankins M, Morris C (2014) Development and reliability of a system to classify the eating and drinking ability of people with cerebral palsy. *Dev Med Child Neurol*, 56, 245–51.

67. Sellers D, Pennington L, Bryant E, et al. (2022) Mini-EDACS: Development of the Eating and Drinking Ability Classification system for young children with cerebral palsy. *Dev Med Child Neurol*, 64, 897–906.

68. Baranello G, Signorini S, Tinelli F, et al. (2020) Visual Function Classification System for children with cerebral palsy: Development and validation. *Dev Med Child Neurol*, 62, 104–110.

69. Paulson A, Vargus-Adams J (2017) Overview of four functional classification systems commonly used in cerebral palsy. *Children*, 4, 1–10.

70. Piscitelli D, Ferrarello F, Ugolini A, Verola S, Pellicciari L (2021) Measurement properties of the Gross Motor Function Classification System, Gross Motor Function Classification System-expanded & revised, Manual Ability Classification System, and Communication Function Classification System in cerebral palsy: A systematic review with meta-analysis. *Dev Med Child Neurol*, 63, 1251–1261.

71. Shevell M (2019) Cerebral palsy to cerebral palsy spectrum disorder: Time for a name change? *Neurology*, 92, 233–35.

72. Holsbeeke L, Ketelaar M, Schoemaker MM, Gorter JW (2009) Capacity, capability, and performance: Different constructs or three of a kind? *Arch Phys Med Rehabil*, 90, 849–55.

73. Rosenbaum P, Gorter JW (2012) The 'f-words' in childhood disability: I swear this is how we should think! *Child Care Health Dev*, 38, 457–63.

74. Gage JR (1991) *Gait analysis in cerebral palsy*, London: Mac Keith Press.

75. Horstmann HM, Bleck EE (2007) *Orthopaedic management in cerebral palsy,* London: Mac Keith Press.

76. Howard J, Soo B, Graham HK, et al. (2005) Cerebral palsy in Victoria: Motor types, topography and gross motor function. *J Paediatr Child Health,* 41, 479–83.

77. Carnahan K, Arner M, Hagglund G (2007) Association between gross motor function (GMFCS) and manual ability (MACS) in children with cerebral palsy. A population-based study of 359 children. *BMC Musculoskelet Disord,* 8, 1–7.

78. Rice J, Russo R, Halbert J, Van Essen P, Haan E (2009) Motor function in 5-year-old children with cerebral palsy in the South Australian population. *Dev Med Child Neurol,* 51, 551–6.

79. Unes S, Tuncdemir M, Ozal C, et al. (2022) Relationship among four functional classification systems and parent interpredicted intelligence level in children with different clinical types of cerebral palsy. *Dev Neurorehabil,* 25, 410–416.

80. Delacy MJ, Reid SM, Australian Cerebral Palsy Register Group (2016) Profile of associated impairments at age 5 years in Australia by cerebral palsy subtype and Gross Motor Function Classification System level for birth years 1996 to 2005. *Dev Med Child Neurol,* 58, 50–6.

81. Hadders-Algra M (2014) Early diagnosis and early intervention in cerebral palsy. *Front Neurol,* 5, 1–13.

82. Keogh J, Sugden DA (1985) *Movement skill development,* London: Macmillan.

83. Day SM, Strauss DJ, Vachon PJ, et al. (2007) Growth patterns in a population of children and adolescents with cerebral palsy. *Dev Med Child Neurol,* 49, 167–71.

84. Brooks J, Day S, Shavelle R, Strauss D (2011) Low weight, morbidity, and mortality in children with cerebral palsy: New clinical growth charts. *Pediatrics,* 128, 299–307.

85. Wright CM, Reynolds L, Ingram E, Cole TJ, Brooks J (2017) Validation of us cerebral palsy growth charts using a uk cohort. *Dev Med Child Neurol,* 59, 933–938.

86. Centers for Disease Control and Prevention (2000a) *2 to 20 years: Girls stature -for-age and weight-for-age percentiles [pdf].* [online] Available at: <https://www.cdc.gov/growthcharts/data/set2clinical/cj41c072.pdf> [Accessed February 22 2024].

87. Centers for Disease Control and Prevention (2009) *Birth to 24 months: Girls length-for-age and weight-for-age percentiles [pdf].* [online] Available at: <https://www.cdc.gov/growthcharts/data/who/GrChrt_Girls_24LW_9210.pdf> [Accessed June 19 2024].

88. Centers for Disease Control and Prevention (2000b) *2 to 20 years: Boys stature-for-age and weight-for-age percentiles [pdf].* [online] Available at: <https://www.cdc.gov/growthcharts/data/set1clinical/cj41l021.pdf> [Accessed February 22 2024].

89. Centers for Disease Control and Prevention (2001) *Birth to 36 months: Boys length-for-age and weight-for-age percentiles [pdf].* [online] Available at: <https://www.cdc.gov/growthcharts/data/set1clinical/cj41l017.pdf> [Accessed February 22 2024].

90. Park ES, Park CI, Cho SR, Na SI, Cho YS (2004) Colonic transit time and constipation in children with spastic cerebral palsy. *Arch Phys Med Rehabil,* 85, 453–6.

91. Murphy KP, Boutin SA, Ide KR (2012) Cerebral palsy, neurogenic bladder, and outcomes of lifetime care. *Dev Med Child Neurol,* 54, 945–50.

92. Azouz H, Abdelmohsen A, Ghany H, Mamdouh R (2021) Evaluation of autonomic nervous system in children with spastic cerebral palsy: Clinical and electophysiological study. *Egypt Rheumatol Rehabil,* 48, 1–9.

93. Nuckolls GH, Kinnett K, Dayanidhi S, et al. (2020) Conference report on contractures in musculoskeletal and neurological conditions. *Muscle Nerve,* 61, 740–744.

94. Kendall FP, McCreary EK, Provance PG, McIntyre Rodgers M, Romani WA (2005) *Muscles: Testing and function with posture and pain,* Baltimore: Lippincott Williams & Wilkins.

95. Hislop HJ, Montgomery J (1995) *Daniels and Worthingham's muscle testing techniques of manual examination,* Philadelphia: WB Saunders.

96. Gage JR, Schwartz MH (2009a) Normal gait. In: Gage JR, Schwartz MH, Koop SE, Novacheck TF, editors, *The identification and treatment of gait problems in cerebral palsy.* London: Mac Keith Press, pp 31–64.

97. Stout JL (2023) Gait: Development and analysis. In: Palisano R, Orlin M, Schreiber J, editors, *Campbell's physical therapy for children 6th edition.* St. Louis: Elsevier, pp 159–183.

98. Gage JR, Novacheck TF (2001) An update on the treatment of gait problems in cerebral palsy. *J Pediatr Orthop,* 10, 265–74.

99. Gage JR, Schwartz MH (2009b) Consequences of brain injury on musculoskeletal development. In: Gage JR, Schwartz MH, Koop SE, Novacheck TF, editors, *The identification and treatment of gait problems in cerebral palsy.* London: Mac Keith Press, pp 107–129.

100. Pollock AS, Durward BR, Rowe PJ, Paul JP (2000) What is balance? *Clin Rehabil,* 14, 402–6.

101. Clauser CE, McConville JT, Young JW (1969) Weight, volume, and center of mass of segments of the human body [pdf] Available at: <https://ntrs.nasa.gov/api/citations/19700027497/downloads/19700027497.pdf> [Accessed June 19 2024].

102. Peterka RJ (2018) Sensory integration for human balance control. *Handb Clin Neurol,* 159, 27–42.

103. Dewar R, Love S, Johnston LM (2015) Exercise interventions improve postural control in children with cerebral palsy: A systematic review. *Dev Med Child Neurol,* 57, 504–20.

104. Lance JW (1980) Pathophysiology of spasticity and clinical experience with baclofen. In: Feldman RG, Young RR, Koella WP, editors, *Spasticity: Disordered motor control.* Chicago: Year Book Medical, pp 183–203.

105. Bohannon RW, Smith MB (1987) Interrater reliability of a modified Ashworth scale of muscle spasticity. *Phys Ther,* 67, 206–7.

106. Numanoglu A, Gunel MK (2012) Intraobserver reliability of modified Ashworth scale and modified Tardieu scale in the assessment of spasticity in children with cerebral palsy. *Acta Orthop Traumatol Turc,* 46, 196–200.

107. Gracies JM, Burke K, Clegg NJ, et al. (2010) Reliability of the Tardieu scale for assessing spasticity in children with cerebral palsy. *Arch Phys Med Rehabil,* 91, 421–8.

108. Barry MJ, Vanswearingen JM, Albright AL (1999) Reliability and responsiveness of the Barry-Albright Dystonia Scale. *Dev Med Child Neurol,* 41, 404–11.

109. Jethwa A, Mink J, Macarthur C, et al. (2010) Development of the Hypertonia Assessment Tool (HAT): A discriminative tool for hypertonia in children. *Dev Med Child Neurol,* 52, 83–7.

110. Knights S, Datoo N, Kawamura A, Switzer L, Fehlings D (2014) Further evaluation of the scoring, reliability, and validity of the Hypertonia Assessment Tool (HAT). *J Child Neurol,* 29, 500–4.

111. Wiley ME, Damiano DL (1998) Lower-extremity strength profiles in spastic cerebral palsy. *Dev Med Child Neurol,* 40, 100–7.

112. Barrett RS, Lichtwark GA (2010) Gross muscle morphology and structure in spastic cerebral palsy: A systematic review. *Dev Med Child Neurol,* 52, 794–804.

113. Modlesky CM, Zhang C (2020) Complicated muscle-bone interactions in children with cerebral palsy. *Curr Osteoporos Rep,* 18, 47–56.

114. Stackhouse SK, Binder-Macleod SA, Lee SC (2005) Voluntary muscle activation, contractile properties, and fatigability in children with and without cerebral palsy. *Muscle Nerve,* 31, 594–601.

115. Theologis T (2013) Lever arm dysfunction in cerebral palsy gait. *J Child Orthop,* 7, 379–82.

116. Kalkman BM, Bar-On L, Cenni F, et al. (2017) Achilles tendon moment arm length is smaller in children with cerebral palsy than in typically developing children. *J Biomech,* 56, 48–54.

117. Bittmann MF, Lenhart RL, Schwartz MH, et al. (2018) How does patellar tendon advancement alter the knee extensor mechanism in children treated for crouch gait? *Gait Posture,* 64, 248–254.

118. Noonan KJ, Farnum CE, Leiferman EM, et al. (2004) Growing pains: Are they due to increased growth during recumbency as documented in a lamb model? *J Pediatr Orthop,* 24, 726–31.

119. Carlon S, Taylor N, Dodd K, Shields N (2013) Differences in habitual physical activity levels of young people with cerebral palsy and their typically developing peers: A systematic review. *Disabil Rehabil,* 35, 647–55.

120. Gough M, Shortland AP (2012) Could muscle deformity in children with spastic cerebral palsy be related to an impairment of muscle growth and altered adaptation? *Dev Med Child Neurol,* 54, 495–9.

121. Nordmark E, Hagglund G, Lauge-Pedersen H, Wagner P, Westbom L (2009) Development of lower limb range of motion from early childhood to adolescence in cerebral palsy: A population-based study. *BMC Med,* 7, 1–11.

122. Smith LR, Chambers HG, Lieber RL (2013) Reduced satellite cell population may lead to contractures in children with cerebral palsy. *Dev Med Child Neurol,* 55, 264–70.

123. Dayanidhi S, Dykstra PB, Lyubasyuk V, et al. (2015) Reduced satellite cell number in situ in muscular contractures from children with cerebral palsy. *J Orthop Res*, 33, 1039–45.

124. Domenighetti AA, Mathewson MA, Pichika R, et al. (2018) Loss of myogenic potential and fusion capacity of muscle stem cells isolated from contractured muscle in children with cerebral palsy. *Am J Physiol Cell Physiol*, 315, 247–257.

125. Barber L, Hastings-Ison T, Baker R, Barrett R, Lichtwark G (2011) Medial gastrocnemius muscle volume and fascicle length in children aged 2 to 5 years with cerebral palsy. *Dev Med Child Neurol*, 53, 543–8.

126. Herskind A, Ritterband-Rosenbaum A, Willerslev-Olsen M, et al. (2016) Muscle growth is reduced in 15-month-old children with cerebral palsy. *Dev Med Child Neurol*, 58, 485–91.

127. Soo B, Howard JJ, Boyd RN, et al. (2006) Hip displacement in cerebral palsy. *J Bone Joint Surg Am*, 88, 121–9.

128. Graham HK, Thomason P, Novacheck TF (2014) Cerebral palsy. In: Weinstein SL, Flynn JM, editors, *Lovell and winter's pediatric orthopedics, level 1 and 2.* Philadelphia: Lippincott Williams & Wilkins, pp 484–554.

129. Hägglund G, Alriksson-Schmidt A, Lauge-Pedersen H, et al. (2014) Prevention of dislocation of the hip in children with cerebral palsy: 20-year results of a population-based prevention programme. *Bone Joint J*, 96-B, 1546–52.

130. Walker K (2009) Radiographic evaluation of the patient with cerebral palsy. In: Gage JR, Schwartz MH, Koop SE, Novacheck TF, editors, *The identification and treatment of gait problems in cerebral palsy.* London: Mac Keith Press, pp 244–259.

131. Wise CH (2015) *Orthopaedic manual physical therapy: From art to evidence,* Philadelphia: F.A. Davis.

132. Koop SE (2009) Musculoskeletal growth and development. In: Gage JR, Schwartz MH, Koop SE, Novacheck TF, editors, *The identification and treatment of gait problems in cerebral palsy.* London: Mac Keith Press, pp 21–30.

133. Staheli LT, Engel GM (1972) Tibial torsion: A method of assessment and a survey of normal children. *Clin Orthop Relat Res*, 86, 183–6.

134. Inman VT, Ralston HJ, Todd F (1981) *Human walking,* Baltimore: Williams & Wilkins.

135. Hägglund G, Pettersson K, Czuba T, Persson-Bunke M, Rodby-Bousquet E (2018) Incidence of scoliosis in cerebral palsy. *Acta Orthop*, 89, 443–447.

136. Willoughby KL, Ang SG, Thomason P, et al. (2022) Epidemiology of scoliosis in cerebral palsy: A population-based study at skeletal maturity. *J Paediatr Child Health*, 58, 295–301.

137. Karaguzel G, Holick MF (2010) Diagnosis and treatment of osteopenia. *Rev Endocr Metab Disord*, 11, 237–51.

138. Finbraten AK, Syversen U, Skranes J, et al. (2015) Bone mineral density and vitamin D status in ambulatory and non-ambulatory children with cerebral palsy. *Osteoporos Int*, 26, 141–50.

139. Rodda JM, Graham HK, Carson L, Galea MP, Wolfe R (2004) Sagittal gait patterns in spastic diplegia. *J Bone Joint Surg Br*, 86, 251–8.

140. Steele KM, Shuman BR, Schwartz MH (2017) Crouch severity is a poor predictor of elevated oxygen consumption in cerebral palsy. *J Biomech,* 60, 170–174.

141. Rethlefsen SA, Blumstein G, Kay RM, Dorey F, Wren TA (2017) Prevalence of specific gait abnormalities in children with cerebral palsy revisited: Influence of age, prior surgery, and Gross Motor Function Classification System level. *Dev Med Child Neurol,* 59, 79–88.

142. Õunpuu S, Gorton G, Bagley A, et al. (2015) Variation in kinematic and spatiotemporal gait parameters by Gross Motor Function Classification System level in children and adolescents with cerebral palsy. *Dev Med Child Neurol,* 57, 955–62.

143. Johnson DC, Damiano DL, Abel MF (1997) The evolution of gait in childhood and adolescent cerebral palsy. *J Pediatr Orthop,* 17, 392–6.

144. Bell KJ, Õunpuu S, Deluca PA, Romness MJ (2002) Natural progression of gait in children with cerebral palsy. *J Pediatr Orthop,* 22, 677–682.

145. Gough M, Eve LC, Robinson RO, Shortland AP (2004) Short-term outcome of multilevel surgical intervention in spastic diplegic cerebral palsy compared with the natural history. *Dev Med Child Neurol,* 46, 91–7.

146. Stout JL, Novacheck TF, Gage JR, Schwartz MH (2009) Treatment of crouch gait. In: Gage JR, Schwartz MH, Koop SE, Novacheck TF, editors, *The identification and treatment of gait problems in cerebral palsy.* London: Mac Keith Press, pp 555–578.

147. Rozumalski A, Schwartz MH (2009) Crouch gait patterns defined using k-means cluster analysis are related to underlying clinical pathology. *Gait Posture,* 30, 155–60.

148. Collins M (2014) Strabismus in cerebral palsy: When and why to operate. *Am Orthopt J,* 64, 17–20.

149. Svedberg LE, Englund E, Malker H, Stener-Victorin E (2008) Parental perception of cold extremities and other accompanying symptoms in children with cerebral palsy. *Eur J Paediatr Neurol,* 12, 89–96.

150. Huff JS, Murr N (2023) *Seizure.* [e-book] Treasure Island, StatPearls Publishing. Available at:National Library of Medicine <https://www.ncbi.nlm.nih.gov/books/NBK430765/> [Accessed February 9 2024].

151. Vinkel MN, Rackauskaite G, Finnerup NB (2022) Classification of pain in children with cerebral palsy. *Dev Med Child Neurol,* 64, 447–452.

152. Dickinson HO, Parkinson KN, Ravens-Sieberer U, et al. (2007) Self-reported quality of life of 8-12-year-old children with cerebral palsy: A cross-sectional European study. *Lancet,* 369, 2171–2178.

153. Colver A, Rapp M, Eisemann N, et al. (2015) Self-reported quality of life of adolescents with cerebral palsy: A cross-sectional and longitudinal analysis. *Lancet,* 385, 705–16.

154. Wright AJ, Fletcher O, Scrutton D, Baird G (2016) Bladder and bowel continence in bilateral cerebral palsy: A population study. *J Pediatr Urol,* 12, 1–8.

155. Wiegerink DJ, Roebroeck ME, Van Der Slot WM, et al. (2010) Importance of peers and dating in the development of romantic relationships and sexual activity of young adults with cerebral palsy. *Dev Med Child Neurol,* 52, 576–82.

156. Wiegerink DJ, Roebroeck ME, Bender J, et al. (2011) Sexuality of young adults with cerebral palsy: Experienced limitations and needs. *Sex Disabil,* 29, 119–128.

157. World Health Organization (1995) The World Health Organization quality of life assessment (WHOQOL): Position paper from the World Health Organization. *Soc Sci Med,* 41, 1403–9.

158. World Health Organization (2022) *Mental health.* [online] Available at: <https:// www.who.int/news-room/fact-sheets/detail/mental-health-strengthening-our -response> [Accessed February 22 2024].

159. Downs J, Blackmore A, Epstein A, et al. (2017) The prevalence of mental health disorders and symptoms in children and adolescents with cerebral palsy: A systematic review and meta-analysis. *Dev Med Child Neurol,* 60, 30–38.

160. Rackauskaite G, Bilenberg N, Uldall P, Bech BH, Ostergaard J (2020) Prevalence of mental disorders in children and adolescents with cerebral palsy: Danish nationwide follow-up study. *Eur J Paediatr Neurol,* 27, 98–103.

161. Lindsay S, McPherson AC (2012a) Experiences of social exclusion and bullying at school among children and youth with cerebral palsy. *Disabil Rehabil,* 34, 101–9.

162. Noritz G, Davidson L, Steingass K, The Council on Children with Disabilities, The American Academy for Cerebral Palsy and Developmental Medicine (2022) Providing a primary care medical home for children and youth with cerebral palsy. *American Academy of Pediatrics,* 150, 1–54.

163. Rosenbaum P, Rosenbloom L, Mayston M (2012) Therapists and therapies in cerebral palsy. In: Rosenbaum P, Rosenbloom L, editors, *Cerebral palsy: From diagnosis to adulthood.* London: Mac Keith Press, pp 124–148.

164. Canchild (2024) *Family-centred service.* [online] Available at: <https://canchild .ca/en/research-in-practice/family-centred-service> [Accessed February 22 2024].

165. Stivers T (2012) Physician-child interaction: When children answer physicians' questions in routine medical encounters. *Patient Educ Couns,* 87, 3–9.

166. Martinek TJ (1996) Fostering hope in youth: A model for explaining learned helplessness in physical activity. *Quest,* 48, 409–421.

167. Jahnsen R, Villien L, Aamodt G, Stanghelle J, Inger H (2003) Physiotherapy and physical activity - experiences of adults with cerebral palsy, with implications for children. *Advances in Physiotherapy,* 5, 21–32.

168. Gillette Children's (2018) *Cerebral palsy road map: What to expect as your child grows [pdf].* [online] Available at: <http://gillettechildrens.org/assets/uploads/ care-and-conditions/CP_Roadmap.pdf> [Accessed February 22 2024].

169. Sackett DL, Rosenberg WM, Gray JA, Haynes RB, Richardson WS (1996) Evidence based medicine: What it is and what it isn't. *BMJ,* 312, 71–2.

170. Academy of Pediatric Physical Therapy (2019) Fact sheet: The ABCs of pediatric physical therapy. [pdf] Wisconsin, APTA, Available at: <https://pediatricapta.org/ includes/fact-sheets/pdfs/FactSheet_ABCsofPediatricPT_2019.pdf?v=2> [Accessed April 24 2024].

171. Agency for Healthcare Research and Quality (2020) The SHARE approach: A model for shared decisionmaking - fact sheet, Available at: <https://www.ahrq.gov/health-literacy/professional-training/shared-decision/tools/factsheet.html> [Accessed February 18 2024].

172. Palisano RJ (2006) A collaborative model of service delivery for children with movement disorders: A framework for evidence-based decision making. *Phys Ther,* 86, 1295–305.

173. Mayston M (2018) More studies are needed in paediatric neurodisability. *Dev Med Child Neurol,* 60, 966.

174. Morris ZS, Wooding S, Grant J (2011) The answer is 17 years, what is the question: Understanding time lags in translational research. *J R Soc Med,* 104, 510–20.

175. Deville C, McEwen I, Arnold SH, Jones M, Zhao YD (2015) Knowledge translation of the Gross Motor Function Classification System among pediatric physical therapists. *Pediatr Phys Ther,* 27, 376–84.

176. Bailes A, Gannotti M, Bellows D, et al. (2018) Caregiver knowledge and preferences for gross motor function information in cerebral palsy. *Dev Med Child Neurol,* 60, 1264–1270.

177. Gross PH, Bailes AF, Horn SD, et al. (2018) Setting a patient-centered research agenda for cerebral palsy: A participatory action research initiative. *Dev Med Child Neurol,* 60, 1278–1284.

178. Wallwiener M, Brucker SY, Wallwiener D, Steering C (2012) Multidisciplinary breast centres in Germany: A review and update of quality assurance through benchmarking and certification. *Arch Gynecol Obstet,* 285, 1671–83.

179. Damiano D, Longo E (2021) Early intervention evidence for infants with or at risk for cerebral palsy: An overview of systematic reviews. *Dev Med Child Neurol,* 63, 771–784.

180. Ogbeiwi O (2018) General concepts of goals and goal-setting in healthcare: A narrative review. *Journal of Management & Organization,* 27, 324–341.

181. Löwing K, Bexelius A, Brogren Carlberg E (2009) Activity focused and goal directed therapy for children with cerebral palsy–do goals make a difference? *Disabil Rehabil,* 31, 1808–16.

182. Phoenix M, Rosenbaum P (2014) Development and implementation of a paediatric rehabilitation care path for hard-to-reach families: A case report. *Child Care Health Dev,* 41, 494–9.

183. Vroland-Nordstrand K, Eliasson AC, Jacobsson H, Johansson U, Krumlinde-Sundholm L (2016) Can children identify and achieve goals for intervention? A randomized trial comparing two goal-setting approaches. *Dev Med Child Neurol,* 58, 589–96.

184. Franki I, De Cat J, Deschepper E, et al. (2014) A clinical decision framework for the identification of main problems and treatment goals for ambulant children with bilateral spastic cerebral palsy. *Res Dev Disabil,* 35, 1160–76.

185. Law M, Baptiste S, Carswell A, et al. (2019) *Canadian Occupational Performance Measure.* Ottawa: COMP Inc.

186. Turner-Stokes L (2009) Goal attainment scaling (gas) in rehabilitation: A practical guide. *Clin Rehabil,* 23, 362–70.

187. Narayanan U, Davidson B, Weir S (2011) The Gait Outcomes Assessment List (GOAL): A new tool to assess cerebral palsy. *Dev Med Child Neurol, 53*, 79.

188. Thomason P, Tan A, Donnan A, et al. (2018) The Gait Outcomes Assessment List (GOAL): Validation of a new assessment of gait function for children with cerebral palsy. *Dev Med Child Neurol, 60*, 618–623.

189. Boyer E, Palmer M, Walt K, Georgiadis A, Stout J (2022) Validation of the Gait Outcomes Assessment List questionnaire and caregiver priorities for individuals with cerebral palsy. *Dev Med Child Neurol, 64*, 379–386.

190. Stout JL, Thill M, Munger ME, Walt K, Boyer ER (2024) Reliability of the Gait Outcomes Assessment List questionnaire. *Dev Med Child Neurol, 66*, 61–69.

191. Elkamil AI, Andersen GL, Hägglund G, et al. (2011) Prevalence of hip dislocation among children with cerebral palsy in regions with and without a surveillance programme: A cross sectional study in Sweden and Norway. *BMC Musculoskelet Disord, 12*, 284.

192. Thomason P, Rodda J, Willoughby K, Graham HK (2014) Lower limb function. In: Dan B, Mayston M, Paneth N, Rosenbloom L, editors, *Cerebral palsy: Science and clinical practice.* London: Mac Keith Press, pp 461–488.

193. World Confederation for Physical Therapy (2024) *What is physiotherapy?* [online] Available at: <https://world.physio/resources/what-is-physiotherapy> [Accessed February 22 2024].

194. Dekkers K, Rameckers EAA, Smeets R, et al. (2020) Upper extremity muscle strength in children with unilateral spastic cerebral palsy: A bilateral problem? *Phys Ther, 100*, 2205–2216.

195. Fowler EG, Ho TW, Nwigwe AI, Dorey FJ (2001) The effect of quadriceps femoris muscle strengthening exercises on spasticity in children with cerebral palsy. *Phys Ther, 81*, 1215–23.

196. Gonzalez A, Garcia L, Kilby J, Mcnair P (2021) Robotic devices for paediatric rehabilitation: A review of design features. *BioMedical Engineering OnLine, 20*, 89.

197. Pin T, Dyke P, Chan M (2006) The effectiveness of passive stretching in children with cerebral palsy. *Dev Med Child Neurol, 48*, 855–62.

198. American Occupational Therapy Association (2024) *Patients & clients: Learn about occupational therapy.* [online] Available at: <https://www.aota.org/about/what-is-ot> [Accessed February 22 2024].

199. Bailes A, Reder R, Burch C (2008) Development of guidelines for determining frequency of therapy services in a pediatric medical setting. *Pediatr Phys Ther, 20*, 194–8.

200. Gillette Children's (2024) *Episodes of care in childhood and adolescence.* [online] Available at: <https://www.gillettechildrens.org/assets/REHA-006_EOC_English.pdf> [Accessed January 19 2024].

201. Novak I, McIntyre S, Morgan C, et al. (2013) A systematic review of interventions for children with cerebral palsy: State of the evidence. *Dev Med Child Neurol, 55*, 885–910.

202. American Council on Exercise (2015) *Physical activity vs. Exercise: What's the difference?* [online] Available at: <https://www.acefitness.org/resources/everyone/blog/5460/physical-activity-vs-exercise-what-s-the-difference/> [Accessed February 22 2024].

203. O'Neil ME, Fragala-Pinkham M, Lennon N, et al. (2016) Reliability and validity of objective measures of physical activity in youth with cerebral palsy who are ambulatory. *Phys Ther*, 96, 37–45.

204. Bjornson K, Fiss A, Avery L, et al. (2019) Longitudinal trajectories of physical activity and walking performance by Gross Motor Function Classification System level for children with cerebral palsy. *Disabil Rehabil*, 42, 1705–1713.

205. Bjornson KF, Zhou C, Stevenson R, Christakis D, Song K (2014) Walking activity patterns in youth with cerebral palsy and youth developing typically. *Disabil Rehabil*, 36, 1279–84.

206. Obeid J, Balemans AC, Noorduyn SG, Gorter JW, Timmons BW (2014) Objectively measured sedentary time in youth with cerebral palsy compared with age, sex, and season-matched youth who are developing typically: An explorative study. *Phys Ther*, 94, 1163–7.

207. Maltais DB, Pierrynowski MR, Galea VA, Bar-Or O (2005) Physical activity level is associated with the O2 cost of walking in cerebral palsy. *Med Sci Sports Exerc*, 37, 347–53.

208. Ryan JM, Hensey O, McLoughlin B, Lyons A, Gormley J (2014) Reduced moderate-to-vigorous physical activity and increased sedentary behavior are associated with elevated blood pressure values in children with cerebral palsy. *Phys Ther*, 94, 1144–53.

209. Slaman J, Roebroeck M, Van Der Slot W, et al. (2014) Can a lifestyle intervention improve physical fitness in adolescents and young adults with spastic cerebral palsy? A randomized controlled trial. *Arch Phys Med Rehabil*, 95, 1646–55.

210. Maher CA, Toohey M, Ferguson M (2016) Physical activity predicts quality of life and happiness in children and adolescents with cerebral palsy. *Disabil Rehabil*, 38, 865–9.

211. Zwinkels M, Verschuren O, Balemans A, et al. (2018) Effects of a school-based sports program on physical fitness, physical activity, and cardiometabolic health in youth with physical disabilities: Data from the sport-2-stay-fit study. *Front Pediatr*, 6, 1–11.

212. Fowler EG, Kolobe TH, Damiano DL, et al. (2007) Promotion of physical fitness and prevention of secondary conditions for children with cerebral palsy: Section on pediatrics research summit proceedings. *Phys Ther*, 87, 1495–510.

213. Verschuren O, Peterson MD, Balemans AC, Hurvitz EA (2016) Exercise and physical activity recommendations for people with cerebral palsy. *Dev Med Child Neurol*, 58, 798–808.

214. World Health Organization (2010) *Global recommendations on physical activity for health.* [online] Available at: <https://www.who.int/publications/i/item/9789241599979> [Accessed February 22 2024].

215. Tipton CM (2014) The history of "exercise is medicine" in ancient civilizations. *Adv Physiol Educ*, 38, 109–17.

216. Adolph KE, Vereijken B, Shrout PE (2003) What changes in infant walking and why. *Child Dev*, 74, 475–97.

217. Loughborough University Peter Harrison Centre for Disability Sport [pdf] (n.d.) *Fit for life*. [online] Available at: <https://www.lboro.ac.uk/media/media/research/phc/downloads/Cerebral%20Palsy%20guide_Fit_for_Life.pdf> [Accessed February 22 2024].

218. Loughborough University Peter Harrison Centre for Disability Sport [pdf] (n.d.) *Fit for sport*. [online] Available at: <https://www.lboro.ac.uk/media/media/research/phc/downloads/Cerebral%20Palsy%20guide_Fit_for_Sport.pdf> [Accessed February 22 2024].

219. World Abilitysport (2024) *World Abilitysport*. [online] Available at: <https://worldabilitysport.org/> [Accessed February 22 2024].

220. O'Sullivan J (2016) '*We all have limits. I am not a disabled athlete, I am a Paralympic athlete.*' [online] Available at: <https://www.irishtimes.com/sport/we-all-have-limits-i-am-not-a-disabled-athlete-i-am-a-paralympic-athlete-1.2787039> [Accessed February 22 2024].

221. Moore J (2016) *Now four Paralympic athletes beat the Olympic gold medal time, perhaps people will stop telling me I can become one too*. [online] Available at: <https://www.independent.co.uk/voices/paralympics-athletes-beat-olympic-gold-medal-time-1500m-race-disability-stop-asking-me-to-become-one-a7245961.html> [Accessed February 22 2024].

222. International Paralympic Committee (2024) *Paralympic sports list*. [online] Available at: <https://www.paralympic.org/sports> [Accessed February 22 2024].

223. World Health Organization (2024a) *Assistive technology*. [online] Available at: <https://www.who.int/news-room/fact-sheets/detail/assistive-technology> [Accessed February 22 2024].

224. Ward M, Johnson C, Klein J, Mcgeary FJ, Nolin W PM (2021) Orthotics and assistive devices. In: Murphy KP, McMahon MA, Houtrow AJ, editors, *Pediatric rehabilitation principles and practice*. New York: Springer publishing company, pp 196–229.

225. Owen E, Rahlin M, Kane K (2023) Content validity of a collaborative goal-setting pictorial tool for children who wear ankle-foot orthoses: A modified Delphi consensus study. *JPO Journal of Prosthetics and Orthotics*, 32, 89–98.

226. Grunt S, Fieggen AG, Vermeulen RJ, Becher JG, Langerak NG (2014) Selection criteria for selective dorsal rhizotomy in children with spastic cerebral palsy: A systematic review of the literature. *Dev Med Child Neurol*, 56, 302–12.

227. Nicolini-Panisson RD, Tedesco AP, Folle MR, Donadio MVF (2018) Selective dorsal rhizotomy in cerebral palsy: Selection criteria and postoperative physical therapy protocols. *Rev Paul Pediatr*, 36, 100–108.

228. Wang KK, Munger ME, Chen BP, Novacheck TF (2018) Selective dorsal rhizotomy in ambulant children with cerebral palsy. *J Child Orthop*, 12, 413–427.

229. Ward ME (2009) Pharmacologic treatment with oral medications. In: Gage JR, Schwartz MH, Koop SE, Novacheck TF, editors, *The identification and treatment of gait problems in cerebral palsy*. London: Mac Keith Press, pp 349–362.

230. Molenaers G, Desloovere K (2009) Pharmacologic treatment with botulinum toxin. In: Gage JR, Schwartz MH, Koop SE, Novacheck TF, editors, *The identification and treatment of gait problems in cerebral palsy*. London: Mac Keith Press, pp 363–380.

231. Multani I, Manji J, Hastings-Ison T, Khot A, Graham K (2019) Botulinum toxin in the management of children with cerebral palsy. *Paediatr Drugs*, 21, 261–281.

232. Shore BJ, Thomason P, Reid SM, Shrader MW, Graham HK (2021) Cerebral palsy. In: Weinstein S, Flynn J, Crawford H, editors, *Lovell and Winter's pediatric orthopaedics* 8th ed. Philadelphia: Wolters Kluwer, pp 508–589.

233. Williams SA, Elliott C, Valentine J, et al. (2013) Combining strength training and botulinum neurotoxin intervention in children with cerebral palsy: The impact on muscle morphology and strength. *Disabil Rehabil*, 35, 596–605.

234. Love SC, Novak I, Kentish M, et al. (2010) Botulinum toxin assessment, intervention and after-care for lower limb spasticity in children with cerebral palsy: International consensus statement. *Eur J Neurol*, 17, 9–37.

235. Molenaers G, Fagard K, Van Campenhout A, Desloovere K (2013) Botulinum toxin A treatment of the lower extremities in children with cerebral palsy. *J Child Orthop*, 7, 383–7.

236. Fortuna R, Horisberger M, Vaz MA, Herzog W (2013) Do skeletal muscle properties recover following repeat onabotulinum toxin A injections? *J Biomech*, 46, 2426–33.

237. Fortuna R, Vaz MA, Sawatsky A, Hart DA, Herzog W (2015) A clinically relevant BTX-A injection protocol leads to persistent weakness, contractile material loss, and an altered mRNA expression phenotype in rabbit quadriceps muscles. *J Biomech*, 48, 1700–6.

238. Mathevon L, Michel F, Decavel P, et al. (2015) Muscle structure and stiffness assessment after botulinum toxin type A injection. A systematic review. *Ann Phys Rehabil Med*, 58, 343–50.

239. Valentine J, Stannage K, Fabian V, et al. (2016) Muscle histopathology in children with spastic cerebral palsy receiving botulinum toxin type A. *Muscle Nerve*, 53, 407–14.

240. Alexander C, Elliott C, Valentine J, et al. (2018) Muscle volume alterations after first botulinum neurotoxin a treatment in children with cerebral palsy: A 6-month prospective cohort study. *Dev Med Child Neurol*, 60, 1165–1171.

241. Schless SH, Cenni F, Bar-On L, et al. (2019) Medial gastrocnemius volume and echo-intensity after botulinum neurotoxin A interventions in children with spastic cerebral palsy. *Dev Med Child Neurol*, 61, 783–790.

242. Tang MJ, Graham HK, Davidson KE (2021) Botulinum toxin A and osteosarcopenia in experimental animals: A scoping review. *Toxins*, 13, 1–13.

243. Krach LE (2009) Treatment of spasticity with intrathecal baclofen. In: Gage JR, Schwartz MH, Koop SE, Novacheck TF, editors, *The identification and treatment of gait problems in cerebral palsy*. London: Mac Keith Press, pp 383–396.

244. Gillette Children's (2013) *Pediatric spasticity management*. St. Paul: Gillette Children's Hospital. Unpublished.

245. Duffy EA, Hornung AL, Chen BP, et al. (2021) Comparing short-term outcomes between conus medullaris and cauda equina surgical techniques of selective dorsal rhizotomy. *Dev Med Child Neurol,* 63, 336–342.

246. Georgiadis AG, Schwartz MH, Walt K, et al. (2017) Team approach: Single-event multilevel surgery in ambulatory patients with cerebral palsy. *JBJS Rev,* 5, 1–14.

247. Langerak NG, Tam N, Vaughan CL, Fieggen AG, Schwartz MH (2012) Gait status 17–26 years after selective dorsal rhizotomy. *Gait Posture,* 35, 244–9.

248. Bolster EA, Van Schie PE, Becher JG, et al. (2013) Long-term effect of selective dorsal rhizotomy on gross motor function in ambulant children with spastic bilateral cerebral palsy, compared with reference centiles. *Dev Med Child Neurol,* 55, 610–6.

249. Munger ME, Aldahondo N, Krach LE, Novacheck TF, Schwartz MH (2017) Long-term outcomes after selective dorsal rhizotomy: A retrospective matched cohort study. *Dev Med Child Neurol,* 59, 1196–1203.

250. Macwilliams BA, Mcmulkin ML, Duffy EA, et al. (2022) Long-term effects of spasticity treatment, including selective dorsal rhizotomy, for individuals with cerebral palsy. *Dev Med Child Neurol,* 64, 561–568.

251. Dreher T, Thomason P, Svehlik M, et al. (2018) Long-term development of gait after multilevel surgery in children with cerebral palsy: A multicentre cohort study. *Dev Med Child Neurol,* 60, 88–93.

252. Rang M (1990) Cerebral palsy. In: Morrissy R, editor, *Pediatric orthopedics.* Philadelphia: Lippincott, pp 465–506.

253. Thomason P, Baker R, Dodd K, et al. (2011) Single-event multilevel surgery in children with spastic diplegia: A pilot randomized controlled trial. *J Bone Joint Surg Am,* 93, 451–60.

254. Vuillermin C, Rodda J, Rutz E, et al. (2011) Severe crouch gait in spastic diplegia can be prevented: A population-based study. *J Bone Joint Surg Br,* 93, 1670–5.

255. McGinley JL, Dobson F, Ganeshalingam R, et al. (2012) Single-event multilevel surgery for children with cerebral palsy: A systematic review. *Dev Med Child Neurol,* 54, 117–28.

256. Van Bommel EEH, Arts MME, Jongerius PH, Ratter J, Rameckers EAA (2019) Physical therapy treatment in children with cerebral palsy after single-event multilevel surgery: A qualitative systematic review. A first step towards a clinical guideline for physical therapy after single-event multilevel surgery. *Ther Adv Chronic Dis,* 10, 1–14.

257. Colvin C, Greve K, Lehn C, et al. (2019) *Evidence-based clinical care guideline for physical therapy management of single event multi-level surgeries (SEMLS) for children, adolescents, and young adults with cerebral palsy or other similar neuromotor conditions [pdf].* [online] Available at: <https://www.cincinnati childrens.org/research/divisions/j/anderson-center/evidence-based-care/ recommendations> [Accessed February 22 2024].

258. Gorton GE, Abel MF, Oeffinger DJ, et al. (2009) A prospective cohort study of the effects of lower extremity orthopaedic surgery on outcome measures in ambulatory children with cerebral palsy. *J Pediatr Orthop,* 29, 903–9.

259. Thomason P, Selber P, Graham HK (2013) Single event multilevel surgery in children with bilateral spastic cerebral palsy: A 5 year prospective cohort study. *Gait Posture,* 37, 23–8.

260. Amirmudin NA, Lavelle G, Theologis T, Thompson N, Ryan JM (2019) Multilevel surgery for children with cerebral palsy: A meta-analysis. *Pediatrics,* 143, 1–18.

261. Molenaers G, Desloovere K, De Cat J, et al. (2001) Single event multilevel botulinum toxin type A treatment and surgery: Similarities and differences. *Eur J Neurol,* 8 Suppl 5, 88–97.

262. Saraph V, Zwick EB, Zwick G, et al. (2002) Multilevel surgery in spastic diplegia: Evaluation by physical examination and gait analysis in 25 children. *J Pediatr Orthop,* 22, 150–7.

263. Schwartz MH, Viehweger E, Stout J, Novacheck TF, Gage JR (2004) Comprehensive treatment of ambulatory children with cerebral palsy: An outcome assessment. *J Pediatr Orthop,* 24, 45–53.

264. Zwick EB, Saraph V, Linhart WE, Steinwender G (2001) Propulsive function during gait in diplegic children: Evaluation after surgery for gait improvement. *J Pediatr Orthop B,* 10, 226–33.

265. Rodda JM, Graham HK, Nattrass GR, et al. (2006) Correction of severe crouch gait in patients with spastic diplegia with use of multilevel orthopaedic surgery. *J Bone Joint Surg Am,* 88, 2653–64.

266. Stout JL, Gage JR, Schwartz MH, Novacheck TF (2008) Distal femoral extension osteotomy and patellar tendon advancement to treat persistent crouch gait in cerebral palsy. *J Bone Joint Surg Am,* 90, 2470–84.

267. Delp SL, Statler K, Carroll NC (1995) Preserving plantar flexion strength after surgical treatment for contracture of the triceps surae: A computer simulation study. *J Orthop Res,* 13, 96–104.

268. Novacheck TF (2024) *Personal communication.*

269. Rutz E, Mccarthy J, Shore BJ, et al. (2020) Indications for gastrocsoleus lengthening in ambulatory children with cerebral palsy: A Delphi consensus study. *J Child Orthop,* 14, 405–414.

270. Mus-Peters CTR, Huisstede BMA, Noten S, et al. (2018) Low bone mineral density in ambulatory persons with cerebral palsy? A systematic review. *Disabil Rehabil,* 41, 2392–2402.

271. Mergler S (2018) Bone status in cerebral palsy. In: Panteliadis CP, editor, *Cerebral palsy: A multidisciplinary approach.* Cham: Springer International Publishing, pp 253–257.

272. Gage JR (2009) General issues of recurrence with growth. In: Gage JR, Schwartz MH, Koop SE, Novacheck TF, editors, *The identification and treatment of gait problems in cerebral palsy.* London: Mac Keith Press, pp 546–554.

273. Majnemer A, Shikako-Thomas K, Shevell MI, et al. (2013) Pursuit of complementary and alternative medicine treatments in adolescents with cerebral palsy. *J Child Neurol,* 28, 1443–1447.

274. Graham HK (2014) Cerebral palsy prevention and cure: Vision or mirage? A personal view. *J Paediatr Child Health,* 50, 89–90.

275. King GA, Cathers T, Polgar JM, Mackinnon E, Havens L (2000) Success in life for older adolescents with cerebral palsy. *Qual Health Res*, 10, 734–49.

276. Wehmeyer ML, Palmer S (2003) Adult outcomes for students with cognitive disabilities three-years after high school: The impact of self-determination. *Education and Training in Developmental Disabilities*, 38, 131–144.

277. Damiano DL (2006) Activity, activity, activity: Rethinking our physical therapy approach to cerebral palsy. *Phys Ther*, 86, 1534–40.

278. United Nations (1990) *Convention on the rights of the child.* [online] Available at: <https://www.ohchr.org/en/instruments-mechanisms/instruments/convention-rights-child> [Accessed February 22 2024].

279. United Nations Educational Scientific and Cultural Organization (2017) *School violence and bullying: Global status report.* [online] Available at: <https://unesdoc.unesco.org/ark:/48223/pf0000246970?posInSet=1&queryId=N-EXPLORE-8864b64c-4b12-445e-a56d-b655a1a86afd> [Accessed February 22 2024].

280. Lindsay S, McPherson AC (2012b) Strategies for improving disability awareness and social inclusion of children and young people with cerebral palsy. *Child Care Health Dev*, 38, 809–16.

281. Tindal SR (2017) Students with mild cerebral palsy in the classroom: Information and guidelines for teachers. *Interdisciplinary Journal of Undergraduate Research*, 6, 70–78.

282. Thomason P, Graham HK (2013a) Rehabilitation of children with cerebral palsy after single-event multilevel surgery. In: Robert Iansek R, Meg M, editors, *Rehabilitation in movement disorders.* Cambridge: Cambridge University Press, pp 203–217.

283. Strauss D, Brooks J, Rosenbloom L, Shavelle R (2008) Life expectancy in cerebral palsy: An update. *Dev Med Child Neurol*, 50, 487–93.

284. World Health Organization (2024b) *Adolescent health.* [online] Available at: <https://www.who.int/health-topics/adolescent-health#tab=tab_1> [Accessed February 22 2024].

285. Liptak GS (2008) Health and well being of adults with cerebral palsy. *Curr Opin Neurol*, 21, 136–42.

286. Centers for Disease Control and Prevention (2020) *Disability and health related conditions.* [online] Available at: <https://www.cdc.gov/ncbddd/disabilityandhealth/relatedconditions.html> [Accessed January 19 2024].

287. Novak I, Walker K, Hunt RW, et al. (2016) Concise review: Stem cell interventions for people with cerebral palsy: Systematic review with meta-analysis. *Stem Cells Transl Med*, 5, 1014–25.

288. Wu YW, Mehravari AS, Numis AL, Gross P (2015) Cerebral palsy research funding from the National Institutes of Health, 2001 to 2013. *Dev Med Child Neurol*, 57, 936–41.

289. Tosi LL, Maher N, Moore DW, Goldstein M, Aisen ML (2009) Adults with cerebral palsy: A workshop to define the challenges of treating and preventing secondary musculoskeletal and neuromuscular complications in this rapidly growing population. *Dev Med Child Neurol*, 51, 2–11.

290. Santilli V, Bernetti A, Mangone M, Paoloni M (2014) Clinical definition of sarcopenia. *Clin Cases Miner Bone Metab*, 11, 177–80.

291. Ni Lochlainn M, Bowyer RCE, Steves CJ (2018) Dietary protein and muscle in aging people: The potential role of the gut microbiome. *Nutrients,* 10, 929.

292. Bauer J, Biolo G, Cederholm T, et al. (2013) Evidence-based recommendations for optimal dietary protein intake in older people: A position paper from the PROT-AGE Study Group. *J Am Med Dir Assoc,* 14, 542–59.

293. Resnick B, Nahm ES, Zhu S, et al. (2014) The impact of osteoporosis, falls, fear of falling, and efficacy expectations on exercise among community-dwelling older adults. *Orthop Nurs,* 33, 277–88.

294. World Health Organization (2023) *Noncommunicable diseases.* [online] Available at: <https://www.who.int/news-room/fact-sheets/detail/noncommunicable -diseases> [Accessed February 22 2024].

295. Rauch J (2018) *The happiness curve: Why life gets better after midlife,* London: Bloomsbury Publishing.

296. Sheridan KJ (2009) Osteoporosis in adults with cerebral palsy. *Dev Med Child Neurol,* 51 Suppl 4, 38–51.

297. Ryan JM, Albairami F, Hamilton T, et al. (2023) Prevalence and incidence of chronic conditions among adults with cerebral palsy: A systematic review and meta-analysis. *Dev Med Child Neurol,* 65, 1174–1189.

298. Thomason P, Graham HK (2009) Consequences of interventions. In: Gage JR, Schwartz MH, Koop SE, Novacheck TF, editors, *The identification and treatment of gait problems in cerebral palsy.* London: Mac Keith Press, pp 605–623.

299. Nooijen C, Slaman J, Van Der Slot W, et al. (2014) Health-related physical fitness of ambulatory adolescents and young adults with spastic cerebral palsy. *J Rehabil Med,* 46, 642–7.

300. Gillett JG, Lichtwark GA, Boyd RN, Barber LA (2018) Functional capacity in adults with cerebral palsy: Lower limb muscle strength matters. *Arch Phys Med Rehabil,* 99, 900–906.

301. Cremer N, Hurvitz E, Peterson M (2017) Multimorbidity in middle-aged adults with cerebral palsy. *Am J Med,* 130, 9–15.

302. Peterson MD, Ryan JM, Hurvitz EA, Mahmoudi E (2015) Chronic conditions in adults with cerebral palsy. *JAMA,* 314, 2303–5.

303. O'Connell NE, Smith KJ, Peterson MD, et al. (2019) Incidence of osteoarthritis, osteoporosis and inflammatory musculoskeletal diseases in adults with cerebral palsy: A population-based cohort study. *Bone,* 125, 30–35.

304. Whitney DG, Alford AI, Devlin MJ, et al. (2019) Adults with cerebral palsy have higher prevalence of fracture compared with adults without cerebral palsy independent of osteoporosis and cardiometabolic diseases. *J Bone Miner Res,* 34, 1240–1247.

305. Van Gorp M, Hilberink SR, Noten S, et al. (2020) Epidemiology of cerebral palsy in adulthood: A systematic review and meta-analysis of the most frequently studied outcomes. *Arch Phys Med Rehabil,* 101, 1041–1052.

306. Morgan P, McGinley J (2014) Gait function and decline in adults with cerebral palsy: A systematic review. *Disabil Rehabil,* 36, 1–9.

307. Thorpe D (2009) The role of fitness in health and disease: Status of adults with cerebral palsy. *Dev Med Child Neurol,* 51 Suppl 4, 52–8.

308. Murphy KP (2010) The adult with cerebral palsy. *Orthop Clin North Am,* 41, 595–605.

309. Opheim A, Jahnsen R, Olsson E, Stanghelle JK (2012) Balance in relation to walking deterioration in adults with spastic bilateral cerebral palsy. *Phys Ther,* 92, 279–88.

310. Ryan JM, Cameron MH, Liverani S, et al. (2019) Incidence of falls among adults with cerebral palsy: A cohort study using primary care data. *Dev Med Child Neurol,* 62, 477–482.

311. Thill M, Krach LE, Pederson K, et al. (2023) *Physical and psychosocial consequences of falls in individuals with cerebral palsy [pdf]* [online] Available at: <https://www.medrxiv.org/content/medrxiv/early/2023/08/21/2023.08.16.23294 077.full.pdf> [Accessed June 20 2024].

312. Boyer ER, Patterson A (2018) Gait pathology subtypes are not associated with self-reported fall frequency in children with cerebral palsy. *Gait Posture,* 63, 189–194.

313. Jahnsen R, Villien L, Aamodt G, Stanghelle JK, Holm I (2004) Musculoskeletal pain in adults with cerebral palsy compared with the general population. *J Rehabil Med,* 36, 78–84.

314. Van Der Slot WM, Nieuwenhuijsen C, Van Den Berg-Emons RJ, et al. (2012) Chronic pain, fatigue, and depressive symptoms in adults with spastic bilateral cerebral palsy. *Dev Med Child Neurol,* 54, 836–42.

315. Rodby-Bousquet E, Alriksson-Schmidt A, Jarl J (2021) Prevalence of pain and interference with daily activities and sleep in adults with cerebral palsy. *Dev Med Child Neurol,* 63, 60–67.

316. Whitney DG, Bell S, Whibley D, et al. (2020) Effect of pain on mood affective disorders in adults with cerebral palsy. *Dev Med Child Neurol,* 62, 926–932.

317. Asuman D, Gerdtham UG, Alriksson-Schmidt AI, et al. (2023) Pain and labor outcomes: A longitudinal study of adults with cerebral palsy in Sweden. *Disabil Health J,* 16, 1–8.

318. Jarl J, Alriksson-Schmidt A, Rodby-Bousquet E (2019) Health-related quality of life in adults with cerebral palsy living in Sweden and relation to demographic and disability-specific factors. *Disabil Health J,* 12, 460–466.

319. Vidart D'egurbide Bagazgoitia N, Ehlinger V, Duffaut C, et al. (2021) Quality of life in young adults with cerebral palsy: A longitudinal analysis of the sparcle study. *Front Neurol,* 12, 1–14.

320. Jahnsen R, Villien L, Stanghelle JK, Holm I (2003) Fatigue in adults with cerebral palsy in Norway compared with the general population. *Dev Med Child Neurol,* 45, 296–303.

321. Lundh S, Nasic S, Riad J (2018) Fatigue, quality of life and walking ability in adults with cerebral palsy. *Gait Posture,* 61, 1–6.

322. McPhee PG, Brunton LK, Timmons BW, Bentley T, Gorter JW (2017) Fatigue and its relationship with physical activity, age, and body composition in adults with cerebral palsy. *Dev Med Child Neurol,* 59, 367–373.

323. Russchen HA, Slaman J, Stam HJ, et al. (2014) Focus on fatigue amongst young adults with spastic cerebral palsy. *J Neuroeng Rehabil,* 11, 1–7.

324. National Institute of Mental Health (2024a) *Depression*. [online] Available at: <https://www.nimh.nih.gov/health/topics/depression> [Accessed February 22 2024].

325. Smith KJ, Peterson MD, O'Connell NE, et al. (2019) Risk of depression and anxiety in adults with cerebral palsy. *JAMA Neurol*, 76, 294–300.

326. Gannotti ME, Gorton GE, 3rd, Nahorniak MT, Masso PD (2013) Gait and participation outcomes in adults with cerebral palsy: A series of case studies using mixed methods. *Disabil Health J*, 6, 244–52.

327. National Institute of Mental Health (2024b) *Anxiety disorders*. [online] Available at: <https://www.nimh.nih.gov/health/topics/anxiety-disorders> [Accessed February 22 2024].

328. Alves-Nogueira AC, Silva N, Mcconachie H, Carona C (2020) A systematic review on quality of life assessment in adults with cerebral palsy: Challenging issues and a call for research. *Res Dev Disabil*, 96, 1–20.

329. Van Der Slot WM, Nieuwenhuijsen C, Van Den Berg-Emons RJ, et al. (2010) Participation and health-related quality of life in adults with spastic bilateral cerebral palsy and the role of self-efficacy. *J Rehabil Med*, 42, 528–35.

330. Schmidt AK, Van Gorp M, Van Wely L, et al. (2020) Autonomy in participation in cerebral palsy from childhood to adulthood. *Dev Med Child Neurol*, 62, 363–371.

331. Pettersson K, Rodby-Bousquet E (2021) Living conditions and social outcomes in adults with cerebral palsy. *Front Neurol*, 12, 1–12.

332. Accenture (2018) *Getting to equal: The disability inclusion advantage [pdf]*. [online] Available at: <https://www.accenture.com/content/dam/accenture/final/a-com-migration/pdf/pdf-89/accenture-disability-inclusion-research-report.pdf> [Accessed February 22 2024].

333. Hayward K, Chen AY, Forbes E, et al. (2017) Reproductive healthcare experiences of women with cerebral palsy. *Disabil Health J*, 10, 413–418.

334. Nieuwenhuijsen C, Van Der Laar Y, Donkervoort M, et al. (2008) Unmet needs and health care utilization in young adults with cerebral palsy. *Disabil Rehabil*, 30, 1254–62.

335. Bagatell N, Chan D, Rauch KK, Thorpe D (2017) "Thrust into adulthood": Transition experiences of young adults with cerebral palsy. *Disabil Health J*, 10, 80–86.

336. Freeman M, Stewart D, Cunningham CE, Gorter JW (2018) "If I had been given that information back then": An interpretive description exploring the information needs of adults with cerebral palsy looking back on their transition to adulthood. *Child Care Health Dev*, 44, 689–696.

337. O'Brien G, Bass A, Rosenbloom L (2009) Cerebral palsy and aging. In: O'Brien G, Rosenbloom L, editors, *Developmental disability and aging*. London: Mac Keith Press, pp 39–52.

338. Hilberink SR, Roebroeck ME, Nieuwstraten W, et al. (2007) Health issues in young adults with cerebral palsy: Towards a life-span perspective. *J Rehabil Med*, 39, 605–11.

339. Ryan JM, Crowley VE, Hensey O, McGahey A, Gormley J (2014) Waist circumference provides an indication of numerous cardiometabolic risk factors in adults with cerebral palsy. *Arch Phys Med Rehabil,* 95, 1540–6.

340. Putz C, Döderlein L, Mertens EM, et al. (2016) Multilevel surgery in adults with cerebral palsy. *Bone Joint J,* 98-b, 282–8.

341. Cassidy C, Campbell N, Madady M, Payne M (2016) Bridging the gap: The role of physiatrists in caring for adults with cerebral palsy. *Disabil Rehabil,* 38, 493–8.

342. Gajdosik CG, Cicirello N (2001) Secondary conditions of the musculoskeletal system in adolescents and adults with cerebral palsy. *Phys Occup Ther Pediatr,* 21, 49–68.

343. Murphy KP (2018) Comment on: Cerebral palsy, non-communicable diseases, and lifespan care. *Dev Med Child Neurol,* 60, 733.

344. Rosenbaum P (2019) Diagnosis in developmental disability: A perennial challenge, and a proposed middle ground. *Dev Med Child Neurol,* 61, 620.

345. Schuh L (2023) *Personal communication.*

346. Imms C, Dodd KJ (2010) What is cerebral palsy? In: Dodd KJ, Imms C, Taylor NF, editors, *Physiotherapy and occupational therapy for people with cerebral palsy: A problem-based approach to assessment and management.* London: Mac Keith Press, pp 7–30.

347. Ryan JM, Allen E, Gormley J, Hurvitz EA, Peterson MD (2018) The risk, burden, and management of non-communicable diseases in cerebral palsy: A scoping review. *Dev Med Child Neurol,* 60, 753–764.

348. Sheridan (2019) *Personal communication.*

349. Louw A, Diener I, Butler DS, Puentedura EJ (2011) The effect of neuroscience education on pain, disability, anxiety, and stress in chronic musculoskeletal pain. *Arch Phys Med Rehabil,* 92, 2041–56.

350. Moseley GL, Butler DS (2015) Fifteen years of explaining pain: The past, present, and future. *J Pain,* 16, 807–13.

351. Gettings J (2019) *Personal communication.*

352. Andraweera ND, Andraweera PH, Lassi ZS, Kochiyil V (2021) Effectiveness of botulinum toxin A injection in managing mobility-related outcomes in adult patients with cerebral palsy: Systematic review. *Am J Phys Med Rehabil,* 100, 851–857.

353. Reynolds MR, Ray WZ, Strom RG, et al. (2011) Clinical outcomes after selective dorsal rhizotomy in an adult population. *World Neurosurg,* 75, 138–44.

354. Peterson MD, Gordon PM, Hurvitz EA (2013) Chronic disease risk among adults with cerebral palsy: The role of premature sarcopoenia, obesity and sedentary behaviour. *Obes Rev,* 14, 171–82.

355. Garber CE, Blissmer B, Deschenes MR, et al. (2011) American College of Sports Medicine position stand. Quantity and quality of exercise for developing and maintaining cardiorespiratory, musculoskeletal, and neuromotor fitness in apparently healthy adults: Guidance for prescribing exercise. *Med Sci Sports Exerc,* 43, 1334–59.

Index

Figures and tables indicated by page numbers in italics.